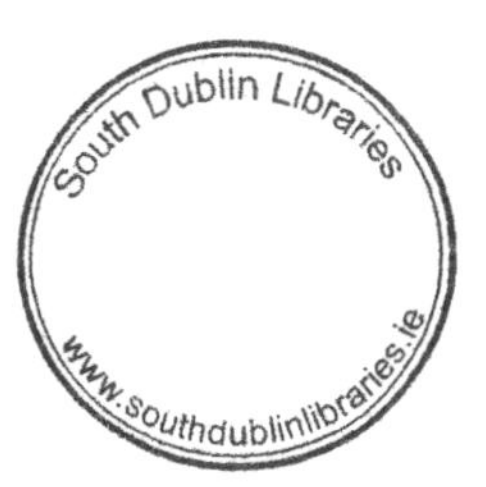

IONBHÁ

THE EMPATHY BOOK FOR IRELAND

IONBHÁ

THE EMPATHY BOOK FOR IRELAND

Edited by

CILLIAN MURPHY, PAT DOLAN,
GILLIAN BROWNE AND MARK BRENNAN

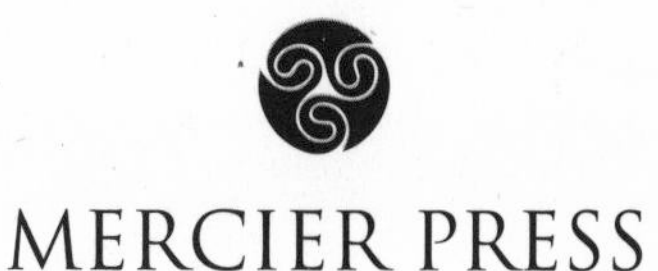

MERCIER PRESS

Dedication

This book is dedicated to all those past, present and future who show empathy, kindness and compassion to others. May we all aspire to this.

MERCIER PRESS
Cork
www.mercierpress.ie

100% of all royalties from the book will go directly to delivering the Activating Social Empathy education programme in Irish schools and youth work organisations.

ISBN: 978-1-78117-819-5

eBook: 978-1-78117-820-1

Cover design: Craig Carry

A CIP record for this title is available from the British Library

Printed and bound in the EU.

Contents

Acknowledgements

The editors wish to acknowledge and thank the following for their support in producing this book: all the contributors who gave so willingly and enthusiastically. The Irish American Partnership for their support in the production and promotion of the book and associated empathy schools programme. Our partners at Foróige deserve acknowledgement for their collaborations with the Activating Social Empathy curriculum. Special thanks to our Youth as Researchers group – Ella Anderson, Jack Gaffey, Róisín Hanley, Caolan Kealy and Mikey Kerin – for their input and thoughtful contributions at all stages of the development of this book. We acknowledge the agents/manager/publicists who helped coordinate many of the contributions included here. Thank you to Craig Carry for his brilliant cover design and for working so diligently with us through all the edits and fine tuning. Thank you to Yvonne McGuinness for her artistic excellence, advice and ideas in the design of the book. All at Mercier Press for their support; *Ollscoil na Gaillimhe* – University of Galway and The Pennsylvania State University for supporting the project.

On Connection

Cillian Murphy

The trick seems to be to work on it. To activate it. To make a connection. To listen. Like learning an instrument, or writing a story ... like a good meditation. All of these things can be taught and can be learnt, and the same is true of empathy.

In 2010, I met Professor Pat Dolan in the Druid Lane theatre in Galway. We immediately fell into a deep conversation about his work at the UNESCO Child and Family Research Centre at *Ollscoil na Gaillimhe* – University of Galway. I was very intrigued by the fact that the centre worked with young people as researchers, that they trained young people in bias and ethics and sent them out to collect data from other young people about their lives and experiences in Ireland. This to me seemed eminently sensible ... that ultimately these findings would be presented to government in order to affect policy in Ireland.

I agreed to become patron for the centre in the hope of promoting that amazing and valuable work, and to help give voice to the work of these resourceful young people. As we continued to work together over the years we began to explore and promote the power of empathy.

At the beginning of this work I was unsure of how to define empathy, or how to locate it in a practical way in my life. I felt that if I was going to promote it, and petition for it to become part of the school curriculum, I needed to understand it.

Slowly as I thought more about it, I began to realise that empathy was actually a fundamental part of my job as an actor. And my job as a Dad.

One of the phrases that you hear over and over as a young actor is 'acting is listening'. This essentially means that you are not truly in a scene unless you are listening and involved and available to everything that your partner in that scene is saying and doing. It sounds easy, but believe me it is not. I speak from experience. As a young actor you are so concentrated on what your character is feeling or experiencing, that you can fail to listen to what other characters are feeling or experiencing …

This is not acting, because there is no connection.

There are many corollaries of this in modern life I guess; the solipsism of social media, the absence of time for others, the echo chamber of the media and politics.

Listening, truly listening, is an empathetic act. Onstage or in film, a banal scene can be elevated to something special when the characters are really listening to each other. The audience feel it.

This must be where the phrase 'a good listener' derives from. We all know instinctively what that means. To be truly heard, to be truly listened to.

So as I continued to work with Pat and everybody at the centre in the University of Galway, I began to learn new things about empathy. That it is different from sympathy … advice is the enemy of empathy.

Empathy is about connection.

I have two sons. Raising boys in this world is difficult. You do everything in your power to avoid raising proto-bullies, to avoid raising proto-misogynists, to avoid all the evil tropes of masculinity we are confronted by everyday.

But I believe kids are naturally empathetic, they might not yet know what that word means, but they have access to it more instinctually than we do as adults. I see this in my own children.

Anything that can encourage this instinct in children is crucial, particularly when they live a good proportion of their lives online, in a competitive and combative atmosphere, where connection is fleeting.

Since 2016 empathy education has been rolled out in schools across Ireland, and offered as part of the curriculum. Activating Social Empathy is a twelve-week empathy training programme, which has been specifically designed for post-primary school students.

The content of programme is structured around four key learning areas (Understanding Empathy; Practising Empathy; Overcoming Barriers to Empathy; Putting Empathy in Action). First, students learn about what empathy is and why it is important; students then spend a number of weeks practising and strengthening their empathy skills; next they spend time discussing the barriers to empathy and brainstorming on how they can overcome these barriers; and finally the programme culminates with students 'putting empathy into action' and taking part in a social action project of their own choosing.

In 2020, the child and family research centre carried out a randomised control trial study on the schools empathy programme. The results were fascinating. Having completed the programme, students showed higher levels of cognitive empathy (e.g. they were better able to understand other people's perspectives) and affective empathy (e.g. they were more willing to share the emotions/feelings of others).

In fact, there is emerging research from neuroscience which shows a positive connection between empathy education in young people and better academic performance – what's been coined as 'firing Gandhi neurons'.

So it exists, and it can be harnessed. It exists in its simplest form as the ability to put yourself into the shoes of another, but it can also be transformed into real positive altruistic action. It can offer an embrace to difference, be a bulwark against intolerance and can bring connection in a disconnected world.

Thank you reader for picking up this book, all proceeds of which will go directly back into the programme you have just been reading about.

In here you will find many and varied reflections on empathy … some very personal, some more objective, some very moving, from people of all walks of life in Ireland. And hopefully you will find some connection.

Unpacking Empathy

Charlotte Silke and Bernadine Brady

In our everyday lives, we encounter things that affect us deeply – for example, hearing about a child who has been bullied, a colleague struggling with ill-health or families fleeing their homes in Ukraine. We find ourselves thinking about these people over and over, trying to imagine what the experience must be like for them, reflecting on how they are feeling and the implications of these events for them. The human emotion of empathy is the reason why.

The term empathy is a relatively new word in the English language. First coined in 1908, empathy is a direct translation of the German word *Einfühlung*, meaning 'feeling-into'. Closely related to concepts such as compassion, sympathy and kindness, empathy is the process of how human beings relate to one another. An essential ingredient in human relationships, empathy refers to our ability to adopt and understand the emotions, feelings and perspectives of others.

Although empathy is one word, it refers to two, separate processes – one relating to our feelings and the other relating to our thoughts. The first component of empathy refers to our ability to share the feelings of others – for example, feeling sad when a friend receives upsetting news. It is important not to confuse this type of response with pity; emotional empathy moves beyond sympathy or pity and involves mirroring the emotions of others – we feel as others feel – as if we are sharing the experience with them. The other part of empathy refers to our ability to understand the emotions and experiences of others – being able to recognise when a friend is disappointed, for example, or being able to understand why someone reacted the way that they did. This aspect of empathy is sometimes referred to as 'perspective taking' or the ability to put yourself in another person's shoes. But an important caveat is that true empathy involves being able to imagine how others feel in their shoes, rather than thinking about how you would feel if you were in those shoes.

Why is empathy important? Empathy is important because it has several notable benefits for individuals and for society. Not surprisingly, when we have higher levels of empathy, our relationships are better. Empathetic people help others more, and crucially, help in a way that is more responsive and attuned to the other person's needs. Empathetic people are happier and get more enjoyment out of life. They show greater resilience to mental illness and stress and have better physical health. As well as helping with the good stuff, empathy helps to prevent the bad stuff. People with higher levels of empathy are less likely to engage in bullying, less likely to act aggressively and less likely to discriminate against others. For these reasons, empathy is seen as essential for the health of democracy and civil society, enabling us to see and respond to the experiences of fellow humans.

Empathy is seen as the great human connector – but where does it come from? We know that empathy is a trait that is both biologically inherited and a skill that can be learned. Children are typically born with an innate capacity for empathy – a trait which appears to be genetically inherited from their parents. In emotional situations, babies as young as 8–10 months will respond automatically with empathy. Infants are not only able to recognise when a person is in distress, but also show concern for that person. Empathy is seen as a trait that is favoured by evolution – we are born with a capacity for empathy, because it increases our chances for survival. Human children need others to care for them, to be able to identify and respond to their needs, and empathy is integral to this.

On the other hand, there is ample evidence to suggest that empathy can be learned (or unlearned). Research shows that by the time children reach adulthood, empathy no longer appears to be an automatic reaction. Although children may be born with an innate tendency for empathy, along the path to adulthood this capacity is strengthened or eroded depending on their environment. In this sense, empathy can be seen as a muscle; we might be born with it, but if we don't use it, practise it, or exercise it, we may lose it. And there is evidence to suggest that this is happening – that in comparison to previous generations, less empathy is being expressed in modern society.

The nature of the modern world can both constrain or enable empathy. For example, much of our social interaction now takes place online. Social media has made it easier for people to share their stories and connect with others in meaningful ways. But it can also be more difficult to empathise with a person behind a screen. With our 24/7 news and celebrity social media feeds, it is not possible to care about every person or group in distress, leading to a phenomenon known as 'empathy fatigue'. There is a human tendency to show greater empathy to people who are close to us or are similar to us and deny empathy to those we see as 'other'. The American sociologist Arlie Hochschild argues that we all unconsciously draw empathy maps, meaning that 'we draw boundaries around high empathy, low empathy and no empathy zones. We feel deeply for the people within a high empathy zone and refuse empathy to those in the no-go zone'. This can happen subconsciously, in that we may not show empathy to others simply because we do not think of them or because we assume that someone else will care about their needs. We have also seen the emergence of populist politics which has nurtured divisions between groups in society, deeming particular groups to be responsible for contemporary problems and therefore unworthy of empathy.

We know from research that there are lots of ways we can help children and young people practise and strengthen their empathy skills. Because the development of empathy is heavily influenced by the culture and environment they grow up in – parents, schools, and friends play an important role in shaping empathy. Simple practices – like parents asking their children to think about how the child they just fought with feels – or being around people who show empathy to others can make a huge difference in nurturing empathy. Learning about social issues and talking about societal problems at school has been shown to help the development of empathy. For all of us, it may be worth reflecting on our own 'empathy maps', thinking about how we can extend our boundaries to bring more people into the high empathy zone, so that we can be more observant and attuned to the needs of all groups and people in society, and not just those who are most like us.

Brothers

Michael D. Higgins

When we set out together to find
our new home,
I suspect
we cared less
for the broken heart of our mother
who had to let us go
than for the wonder of the journey
in a black Ford Eight
through fields
at twilight.

It is that wonder
that brings me back
to the age of five,
not any great grief
I should have felt
or tears I should have shed.

And then, we were
together,
a source of curiosity,
a legacy from tragedy
that had given a childless pair,
an uncle and an aunt,
two instant children,
brothers
so alike

we could be twins.
That's what they said.
We did not find
the bonding
of such words
a burden.

We stood together in photographs.
Our teeth defined
a hidden difference
and, on our city visits,
both wearing boots
for the lasting,
not shoes,
which we were told by our mother
were the mark
of civilisation
and the city,
our Communion suits, chosen
for next year's wear,
the sleeves
played with our knuckles,
another country sign
that made her sad.

At night we shared a prayer
in a room
demoted from a parlour
to being the sleeping place
of aunt and child,
of uncle and child,
the parlour now the space

of what had once been
a four-poster bed,
a sofa and sister bed,
a well-sprung inheritance of iron,
replete with tick and bolster.
We learned those country words,
the rites of night
and intimacy.

Their shaking preceding our prayers,
'Matthew, Mark, Luke and John,
bless this bed that I lay on.'
Evangelists.
I learned the word
and thought of bells
and books
and quills
and long grey beards.

I placed them nightly
on the missing poles
of the bed, mutilated
without its postered canopy,
acquired from the scattering
of a half-great local house.

And the little things were made
for the little men
who would one day be sure
to be a great help
when needed in hayfields
and the bog

or in the wet brown drills
of tillage.

You were better at all these
practical tests
of strength
and judgement too.
For me, the image of escape,
distracted
from the tasks of place.
The books I loved
were instruments
for the breaking of the bars
and a run towards the light
and a new life
back
in the city.

At times, on the bar of a bike,
I vowed
to bring you
where I presumed
you wished to go.

It was through pain
I realised
that our journeys
would be separate,
alone,
requiring different skills

And I sought my brother

in a hundred others
for whom
my heart warmed
at shared
hopes
and fears.

Every embrace a compensation
for the lost moments
of feelings
buried beneath
the boulders
of other expectations
of duty
and respectability
of fear
and dust
and sweat
and a life reduced
to rehearsal
for the decency in death
that was the legacy
of our family.

Back from the tomb,
Christ saw brothers
everywhere.
The stone rolled back,
he never returned
home
but embraced every stranger,
brothers all,

in the light,
out of the dark.

The Talker

Rory O'Neill

I'm a talker. By nature, I'm a talker. And it's a trait for which I'm often grateful. I might be at some kind of 'do' and suddenly everyone is looking at me expecting me to say a few words, and I wasn't expecting to have to say a few words – but it's grand, sure it's only talking.

And sometimes it's even a trait of mine for which other people are grateful. Like some time ago when a friend of mine had a party. It wasn't a formal party, but it wasn't like any of the parties she'd previously had, which were all decided upon spontaneously at 2 a.m. on the pavement outside the pub, and which invariably included a long discussion at 5 a.m. about who was going to go down to the petrol station to get cigarettes and maybe some Rancheros, if they have any. This was her first proper party, in her first home, and she'd invited not just her mate-mates, but also some work mates, and (because she's an idiot sometimes) her new neighbours on both sides. This was the first time she'd ever had a party with a suggested arrival time. She got finger foods from Marks & Spencer!

I arrived a bit earlier than I had planned and when she opened the door and saw me – this woman who knows me well and knows I'm a talker – she just pointed towards the living room and ran back into the kitchen without saying a word. She didn't have to, because the flicker of relief on her stressed face when she saw it was me, and the slight hint of burned M&S prawn puff pastry thingies in the air, told me everything I needed to know. 'Grand, I'm on it!' I said pointlessly because she was already gone, and I opened the living room door to where a handful of other early arrivals were standing around in awkward silence, each of them apparently fascinated by the exquisite craftsmanship of the Tesco wine glasses they were holding, and each of them praying I was someone they knew. I wasn't but it didn't matter because 'My God! I can't believe the size of that new development down the end of the road! And it's like it appeared overnight. Isn't that where the Spar used to be? I always liked that Spar for some reason!' And I was very interested in how they all felt about the now lost Spar, and where she had picked up those beautiful earrings.

Yes I'm a talker and sometimes glad of it. And I come from a family of talkers, and I'm also glad of that, because ironically they're not shy about telling you to shut up and listen sometimes. Because in a family of talkers you learn quickly that if everyone is talking and nobody is listening, it's just a lot of noise. Listening and talking are both important life skills, and even if you have a natural gift for one or the other, you still have to practise it. And it's unlikely you have a gift for both, so at the very least you have to learn one and practise both.

Because you need both. You need one to tell, and the other to hear.

You need one to able to tell your story, and the other to hear other people's stories. And that's important because it's in the telling and hearing of people's stories that empathy is born. And empathy, in the humble opinion of this human, is the most important of all our human attributes. The ability to empathise, the ability to put yourself in someone else's shoes, to be able to imagine yourself in their skin, is the difference between being merely a human mammal, and being a person. Empathy is at the root of all our best qualities – kindness, generosity, fairness, charity, care, love, compassion.

And an inability to feel empathy is a trait common to all psychopaths.

Through the Eyes of Another

Pamela Joyce

Growing up I had no awareness of the word empathy. I didn't know its definition. Thankfully, it was for a good reason. Without knowing it, I had been shown so much empathy throughout my life that I had no reason to believe there was anything else. My family and friends are all empaths. The same goes for my teachers, my neighbours, my sports coaches. In my twenty-eight years, I feel very privileged to say that I have been exposed to empathy time and time again.

It was only when I reached my early to mid twenties that I became accustomed with the word. Not through any one major event but as part of the trials and tribulations of growing up. As you get a bit older, people tend to stop letting you get away with things – the follies of youth don't apply as much anymore. And the same goes for empathy. There is an unspoken rule that at a certain stage in your life you must simply begin to 'get on with things' and 'play the hand you are dealt'. Which I can't say I agree with.

There is always space for empathy.

It is only now in my late twenties that I can fully appreciate the words of Atticus Finch in Harper Lee's *To Kill a Mockingbird:*

'You never really understand a person until you consider things from his point of view ... until you climb into his skin and walk around in it.'

My teacher could not stress enough how important this quote was as a testament to the type of man Atticus was. I must have written that quote in every single essay I wrote in Junior Cert without truly appreciating its meaning.

Yet it is not just Atticus Finch who is a shining beacon of empathy when it comes to fictional characters. X-Men's Professor X embodies all the traits of an empath – most notably the desire to help those in need. Jedi Master Yoda sat in the swampy marshes of Dagobah and trained a young Luke Skywalker, at his own expense. Even the halls of Hogwarts are teaming with empaths in the form of Hufflepuffs. I will admit that as a Ravenclaw I used to turn my nose up at Hufflepuffs – not anymore.

For empathy is a subtle trait. It's not the same as being a muscular hero or an undeniably beautiful person. Your empathy probably won't land you on the front page of a newspaper. And is unlikely you will have suitors banging down your door to get a glimpse of your empathy. Yet this does not diminish its strength. Kindness is at the core of empathy. Allowing yourself to feel something for someone else in an attempt to better understand them.

We all go through struggles in life and it is the people around us and their empathy that helps us navigate these stormy waters. For a long time I found it hard to differentiate between 'empathy' and 'sympathy'. I have tried as best as I can to give you my definition of empathy in the poem below. So in all that you do, I implore you to be an empath.

In life there are, so many things, that lift you up,
and give you wings

A smile, a laugh, a playful wink,
that make you pause, and start to think
To think about, how people care, and how they feel,
about what you share
And if you're lucky, they will be,

the personification, of empathy

They'll understand, your point of view, and realise,
what you're going through

It may be big,
it may be small,
but they will help you, through it all

So take the time, to appreciate, and in return, reciprocate

A friend might share, they're feeling low, above all else
let empathy show

A family member, might need your hand, just let them
know
you understand

When empathy, is who you are, to others,
you're a shining star

A source of hope, where there was none, that you have
changed, by being One

One of those who listens, and is never there to judge,
One who hears them, warts and all, and will never hold
a grudge

One who gives them guidance, when they are in a rut,
without the fear of hearing, 'so what?' or 'tut tut tut'

So when life gives someone lemons, you now know what
to do,
join them in making lemonade, and let empathy shine
through.

Sausage Poisoning

Blindboyboatclub

In the village of Wibald Germany, in 1793, there was an outbreak of food poisoning that killed thirteen people. Their eyelids drooped, their muscles became limp, their facial muscles froze. They had eaten blutwurst. The congealed blood of an animal encased in its gut and boiled. Their disease became known as Sausage Poisoning.

Empathy is a skill that I have learned over the years. It's not an instinct or a gut reaction for me. It's a tool that I've had to develop through mindful awareness and self-compassion. When I was nineteen. I suffered from anxiety attacks. Mine were an intense, incredibly real sensation of panic accompanied by the belief that I was in the process of dying. Very sudden, and with no warning. Usually in public places. I didn't understand what they were or why they happened. So I blamed the public places and avoided visiting them. I stayed in my bedroom. Surrounded by music, books and objects that interested me. I took comfort in Things and ideas, not people. I became agoraphobic.

With persistent anxiety, it became difficult to label and name my individual emotions. All of my emotions threaded into one great curtain of dread. I just felt 'bad', all of the time, and I wanted to escape that overwhelming bad feeling. Any attempt to put a name on what I was experiencing, or why I was feeling that way, made the curtain heavier and more confusing. It darkened my brain. It took my clarity. I wanted to leave my body, because my body was my enemy. I couldn't identify the shame, fear and the anger that constituted this curtain of dread.

Around this time, I bought a book called *Emotions Revealed* by Paul Ekman. It was a book about human emotions, how to understand emotions and how to recognise them in other people. When I paged through it, I did what we all do when we get a new book. I went to that bit in the middle with the pictures. There were several black and white photos of human faces. Each face bore an expression, and I had to guess the corresponding emotion to that expression. It was a solemn Where's Wally, except Wally was a feeling, and the crowd I had to find him in was human skin and teeth. There was the angry person, their eyes focused so intensely and accusatory that they jumped off the page. Lips curled and teeth snarling. That was the easy one. The other was fear. A person with wide startled eyes and frozen muscles around the mouth. I could identify that one too. I knew fear because I lived with it. I knew anger because I feared the world and the people in it. But as the faces progressed in their subtlety. It became more difficult for me to match the individual expressions with their corresponding human emotion. Is this person startled or joyful? What does that raised eyebrow mean? What's the craic with their lips? Do they like me or do they want me to leave? I couldn't do it. I would try to identify the emotions on the more complex human expressions and would be met with crushing disappointment when I'd confuse contempt for disgust, or happiness for excitement. My anxiety had left me unable to decipher what other humans were feeling.

With anxiety comes shame. The shame of being frightened all of the time. The shame of not knowing why I am frightened, or what I'm frightened of. The shame of being afraid to tell another person that this was my experience of being alive. The shame of the helplessness that accompanies anxiety. The shame of feeling weak, different and incapable. This shame led me to depression.

I'd spend a lot of time watching a dvd of the film *Blade*

Runner. It was set in the far future of 2019. The neon lights snaking through big steamy desolate rain, the sombre synthesized soundtrack and the loneliness of it all. It would bring me calm. When I watched *Blade Runner*, I could wrap my body in the curtain of dread for an hour and feel something that replicated normality. I would relate to Harrison Ford, alone in his darkened apartment, drinking whiskey and using a photo-scanning machine that we'd now call a laptop.

Harrison Ford was a Blade Runner, he hunted androids called replicants who looked exactly like humans in every way except for their absence of innate humanity. A replicant was identified with a Voight Kampff test. An intrusive metal machine that scanned the eyes and the face while the subject was asked questions about their relationships with people and animals. It was an empathy test. If the subject failed the test, then that meant they had no empathy. They were not human, but a replicant, deserving of an immediate and violent death. However, the beauty of *Blade Runner*, is that Harrison Ford himself is a replicant. But he doesn't know it. He's under the illusion that he's a human. He thinks he has empathy. But all of his memories are implanted, his identity and sense of self is a false construct.

When I couldn't correctly match the emotions with the faces in that book, I'd feel like a replicant. An inhuman robot who couldn't tell what another person was feeling from a photo of their face. Not worthy of existing in society. I very unfairly told myself that this is why I enjoyed Blade Runner. I'd constructed a myth about myself. That I was relating to a replicant who spent his spare time in a lonely room and convincing himself he was a human, a fake human with no empathy.

In the village of Wibald Germany, in 1793, there was an outbreak of food poisoning that killed thirteen people. Their eyelids drooped, their muscles became limp, their facial muscles froze. They had eaten blutwurst. The congealed blood of an animal encased in its gut and boiled. Their disease became known as Sausage Poisoning. The sausages contained Botulinum. A toxin that causes the muscles to paralyse. Botulinum is known to us today as Botox. It is used in cosmetic surgery to prevent wrinkles, to keep us looking youthful. But a Botox injection to the face comes at a price. It blocks the nerve signals to the skin and prevents wrinkles from developing. At the expense of comfortably expressing facial emotions. A person who has received a botox injection doesn't frown or smile with ease. In 2001 *The Journal of Emotion and Cognition* published the study 'When did her smile drop? Facial mimicry and the influences of emotional state on the detection of change in emotional expression'. The study focused on the capacity to experience empathy in people who had received botox injections. Empathy is a feeback loop. When you identify that another person is smiling or laughing, we mirror that persons facial expressions and experience a similar emotion. This is empathy. Individuals who had botox injections were unable to mirror another person's emotional state with the muscles of their face. And over time, their capacity to empathise diminished.

In my personal journey, it worked both ways. How could I possibly identify another person's feelings, or read another person's facial expressions, when I myself couldn't identify and label my own emotions? All I knew on a daily basis was the curtain of dread. I felt fear, I felt terror. But not much else. So I began to meditate twice a day. When I meditated, I felt a momentary calm. The curtain of dread was lifted. The fear wasn't present. And I was free to sit with my body and my feelings in a mindful and safe way. Slowly, I turned my concentration inward. I unfolded the fear and found shame underneath. I found anger,

I found jealousy, I found contempt. I found helplessness. A belief about myself that I was incapable of being an autonomous adult who could stand on their own two feet. And a jealousy for other people who could. The curtain of dread started to flutter and I could see through my window. I began to silently observe and identify the full palette of my internal emotional world. By understanding, feeling and identifying my emotions I then began to calmly and safely identify the emotions of others. I'd do it mindfully. The wrinkle of a smile. The raise of an eyebrow in surprise. The furrow of disappointment. The forced teethy smile that masks discomfort. I didn't view other people through the threatening lens of fear that a state of anxiety demands. Anxiety had a way of flooding my experience of the world so that everything and every other person was frightening and harmful. I began to experience empathy. I felt self-compassion, forgiveness for myself. A love for the child in me. I wasn't a non human replicant.

Empathy

Michael Kerin

What is Empathy?

Empathy is what people experience in their life. This is when a person who has the ability to understand how people would feel/experience hard things in their life. It can be a loss of a friend/parent/family member or just having a bad day.

What are the three types of Empathy?

1) Emotional
2) Compassionate
3) Cognitive

Emotional

Emotional empathy is where people share the same personal feelings as if it is their own and being able to connect with these feelings to understand the person's experience/getting to know what that person is going through. Other emotions can be love, sadness or happiness. You can make friends by applying this type of empathy.

Compassionate

Compassionate empathy is where people feel bad about other people's failures or difficulties in their life. It is also the ability/knowledge of what people do experience and to be able to share the same feelings or understandings of each other.

Cognitive

Cognitive empathy is the reaction/response of what other people experience in their life or to something that had happened. It is also the ability to understand or learn from different people's experiences or opinions. You can improve this by applying this type of empathy, in order to understand what they experienced. It can also become a skill-set/talent/ability to understand about other people experiences.

Me and My Life

When I was young, I was born with a disability called Down Syndrome. As I grew older, it didn't affect me as much as it did with other people who had developed problems with it, such as intellectual, physical and medical. Intellectual has to do with the mind and behaviour. Physical has to do with movement or blind and deaf. Lastly medical, is about what happens to your organs which are in your digestion system.

I was born in a place called Hull, which is in Yorkshire, England. I grew up with an Irish upbringing as my parents are Irish. One from Clare and the other from Tipperary. I still consider myself both Irish and English. I have one younger brother called Eoin. My hobbies mostly consist of reading books, music, singing, colouring, watching movies, pets, walks, swimming, clothes, cologne and lastly table tennis. I'm a charity and a community person, where I help charities that need help to improve as a community and as a charity. There are charities that help people in need of assistance. Some examples of this are Vincent de Paul and Down Syndrome Ireland.

I have experienced empathy when in primary, secondary school, family, taking part in community and social outings.

When in primary and secondary school, I had to learn to do what I'm told, to have manners, doing homework and to understand others (for example the teachers). I do get on well with others because I do what I'm told and make friends through it. In both primary and secondary school. I did enjoy being back with school friends, which is important. I know that I didn't enjoy doing the homework and the exams, I just did it, as I didn't think about it or doubting myself to do it. I would have that confidence. Empathy has helped me throughout this, as it helped me to do what I'm told, to have manners and to have a high regard for them as they helped me to pass the subjects.

Outside of school and education, I would be more of a family person that enjoys the company of his parents and family friends and doing things with them. I would value family, over other things because I don't know what I would do without them. Family is important for me because without them me and my brother wouldn't be here in the first place. Empathy has helped me to look out for my younger brother and to help my parents and I realise this.

Taking part in community has helped me to understand other people in what they do and what roles they tend to take on as part of taking part in society and empathy has assisted me to realise this because it is important to help people who need it and who are looking for it, which helps them to achieve the things that are important to them. This is an important factor for others because it will make communities and societies become a close-knitted team. This will result into a big and popular 'empathy' thing for people who get a great satisfaction from doing it, to help others to achieve a common goal/achievement that they would have in common. This gives them happiness in their own life, which is also important too.

Taking part in social outings has helped me to understand other people in what they do in the social events and what roles they tend to take on as a part of taking part of society. Empathy has assisted me to realise it, because it is important to help people who need it and who are looking for it, which helps them to achieve the things that are important to them. This will make communities and societies a close knitted family or team. This results in people doing more things together as a team, which gives them good communication skills, so that, they can apply this to other things such as family or their own personal friends which gives them a great satisfaction of doing it, to help others to achieve a common goal/achievement that they would have in common with.

Empathy has helped me to realise the above-mentioned headings of primary, secondary school, family, taking part in community and social outings. It has helped me to value my education, family and being free to enjoy different things. I have empathy to thank. Thanks empathy.

Thoughts on Empathy's Place in Music

Hozier

Human beings have a remarkable (and at times forgivable) need to find something of themselves in the world around them. It comes naturally to them, but where art and music are concerned, it is a predisposition we can for the most part be grateful for. The stories of love, loss, labour, and hardship that we regularly hear in songs resonate within us our own experiences of the same. We find ourselves in these tales, and as such are gifted a moment in which something otherwise privately experienced (contributing to our sense of alienation) is not only being recognised, preserved and honoured from an outside source – but is being done in a medium cherished and celebrated by society.

With the ever-increasing commodification of artists and their songs, it is important to acknowledge the simple yet transcendent exchange that can take place when a song enters into and touches the hearts of others. The emotional and social function of a song is, to me, tied deeply to the concepts of empathy and of the collective.

Something that might demonstrate this is the fact that all songs rely almost entirely on the presence of the other. The song is written or generated to represent and express something, and is sung outward for the benefit of someone else's enjoyment, enlightenment or preservation. Like most art, the work is given life by sources outside of the artist's mind. However, it is my belief that songs are only truly offered their wings when they find their way into the active musical vocabulary of another person. That is, when they have transmigrated not only into the ears and hearts of others, but their own throats also. There are few art forms where the audience can engage so completely with the art and the performer; intellectually, emotionally and (while singing) physically.

The song, when sung, connects and elevates at once the listener, the singer and the subject together and the collective experience is one that invites all comers. The listener is compelled to join in on the song and in doing so quite literally becomes the singer, while the subject is suspended within and between all present. Through that, the song is offered the new wings I mention above, and ascends to another plain where it can hope to take a sip of that elevated atmosphere reserved only for the likes of poetry, which is, in the starkly beautiful words of Robert Pinsky 'an art in which the medium is the audience's body'. In what might offer a nice thought, a study from the Sahlgrenska Academy at Gothenburg University in Sweden a few years ago observed how communal singing also leads to a synchronisation not just of breath, but of the heart beat also.

Scotland's waulking songs are a good example of how song can develop and operate as a function of the collective, elevating all involved. The songs themselves functioned to accompany the work of preparing cloth, and maintain a flow and steady pace that synchronised the group's rhythm, kept spirits high and mades easier the preparing of the textile. Non-lyrical phrases, not unlike those found elsewhere in mouth-music, would be added to accentuate the rhythmic patterns, but importantly, the group would also sing about their community. Stories from their locale might feature or the group would improvise verses to contain each other's names as they worked. This could be for the purpose of humour, or the purpose of preserving and honouring one another's stories.

When we listen to folk music, we are often brought into tales which may have bounced around the world for centuries, changed in melody and lyric but nearly always maintain a core element of the story or human experience they were generated to represent. As with all story telling, it is this unconscious drive to recognise and honour our own humanity that makes music so universally celebrated and accessible.

I believe it is for this reason I come back to folk music and it's adjacent genres so often. It is a tradition based nearly entirely on the sharing, preserving, and careful handling of the stories of human beings. It is also why I believe the musical forms most closely related to it are as iconic and universally enjoyed as they are. As we know, each generation finds itself in the work of artists like Bob Dylan and Joni Mitchell, etc. So much has been written on this and will be written again but I would simply like to offer one other example of active empathy from a musical style I had the benefit of growing up listening to from a young age, the Blues.

In a much-treasured recording taken on the American holiday of Thanksgiving in 1973, the legendary Blues musician B.B. King played to an audience of prison inmates outside New York City. Apart from it being a stormer of a performance and valuable document, it also offers examples of the different dimensions of empathy that can be at play in any musical performance. B.B King's first words to address the audience are full of an awareness and sensitivity 'I bet a lot of you folks have the blues already …' '… I've come to swap some with you'. He playfully explains to the inmates (much to their enjoyment) that as it turned out, a member of his band was very familiar with many of those working and detained in the prison, and proudly states how that fact made him '… happy, because he works with me'. The crowd welcomes this acknowledgement of their value.

B.B. King eventually launches into the line 'I've been down-hearted, ever since the day we met'. It is a love song, about a man who feels as though his efforts have come to nought, and whose love and dedication has been cast aside and overlooked. Through the song the gradual warming of the crowd reaches fever pitch with each line that they feel witnesses their experience in some way. Although the lyrical content is very much of its time, the classic 'How Blue Can You Get', returns to the refrain 'Our love is nothing but the blues' and although in 2022 it may read like a clichéd blues line, it does speak to a deep wisdom of blues music. To love is to suffer, it is to worry. It is to be vulnerable to hurt, and open to rejection. The risk of opening ones' arms or ones' heart only to have them remain empty is a universal one. All of us will try and fail and suffer pain as a result.

Apart from the creation of a moment in time in which the listener's experience can feel witnessed, the song also provides another valuable function. In its writing and its singing, the song offers a space where the writer or artist's own pain can be named, aired and honoured. Many studies have shown that by bringing ourselves to recognise our own suffering with compassion, we can overcome our challenges far easier and lead happier and more mentally healthy lives. The practise of offering ourselves compassion also makes it easier to offer it to others in turn.

A vital element in song-writing to me, therefore, is honesty and humility. Dishonesty in sharing the depth of our experience does a disservice to the song, its subject and the listener. As my teen idol, Tom Waits once said, 'the world is a hellish place, and bad writing is destroying the quality of our suffering. It cheapens and degrades the human experience, when it should inspire and elevate.'

But it is not just in early and mid-twentieth century recordings that we find iconic articulations of these universalities. Modern pop music still ignites within us that which is commonly yearned for, privately enjoyed, or suffered silently. The phenomenal success of a song like that of 'Good For U' by Olivia Rodrigo speaks to the unavoidable devastation of young love spurned. At the time of this writing, short tik-tok videos are made in the thousands by people of all ages reinterpreting, dueting, reappropriating or otherwise covering the lines of that song. It is not by accident that a sentiment along the lines of 'you look happy and healthy, not me, if you ever cared to ask', speaks to so many. No one is spared the need to have their pain witnessed in some way. The existence of that song offers a place where that need can, on some level, feel met.

The individual cries out for empathy in its own ways, and yearns for an acknowledgement of its sorrows and joys. Regardless of genre, style or era music offers a function where a human being can feel less alone. Even in music devoid of lyrical narrative, the human mind finds a way to project itself into soundscapes and abstract pieces. As social creatures, that sense of connectedness is essential to our mental and, for lack of a better term, spiritual health. We are forever drawn to that space offered by song, where so many of these connections can happen in so easy and natural a way that, in the words of Seamus Heaney in the poem 'At the Wellhead' (about listening to his blind neighbour singing), we partake in an experience that is 'intimate and helpful, like a cure/You didn't notice happening'. In these increasingly difficult times, it's no wonder that people seek to self administer that gentle cure in unprecedented and accelerating numbers.

Toss the Bobbin

Nicola Joyce

The sun rose in the morning, went down at its own pace
And the women of Headford made lace

Honor is my name
And I work these hands with pride
From across the lake now my family's by my side
And I make my living here
A few pennies at a time

Mary is my name
They call me widow since he died
Every days the same I lay flowers by his side
And in the evening I make lace
For a few pennies at a time

And I sing
Toss the bobbin and around the pin
These hands will work to feed our kin
Toss the bobbin and around the pin
Steady moving as I sing

Margaret is my name
And I work these hands with pace
The merchants come around they hardly pay me for my lace
Still I work so carefully
For a few pennies at a time

And I sing toss the bobbin and around the pin
These hands will work to feed our kin
Toss the bobbin and around the pin
Steady moving as I sing

Catherine is my name
The girls all call me Kate
I meet them every day with our bobbins and our lace
And we keep each other strong
And we know that we'll be fine
Because there's laughter and there's song
And a few pennies at a time

The sun rose in the morning
Went down at its own pace
And the women of Headford made lace

I was invited to contribute to this book because of a song I wrote. I come from Headford in County Galway. An intriguing history of our women has been recently uncovered and The Whileaways were asked to document this in song. Headford has a tradition of bobbin lacemaking, highly unusual in Ireland, that dates back to the mid eighteenth century. It was introduced by the women of the St George family, who were landlords in the town. Notwithstanding her own fortunate circumstances, Mrs St George recognised the plight of her tenants and set up the industry in an effort to alleviate poverty. In times of hardship and destitution, hundreds of women turned their hands to the delicate art of bobbin lacemaking to feed their families. The industry thrived through the nineteenth century and supported the town through famine and unrest. It faded away at the beginning of the twentieth century, along with almost any trace of its existence. Lacemaking has historically been by the poor, for the rich, and those who made it rarely celebrated even though whole lives were spent making these intricate, laborious, beautiful pieces. The lacemakers would never get to wear the work of their hands. It would instead adorn the petticoats of some faraway wealthy stranger while the lacemakers were paid a pittance on which they managed to feed their children. Somehow, the fact that Headford lace ever existed was written out of local history and the struggles and triumphs of the resilient women who made it cast aside not as heroic, but irrelevant. The irrelevant work of poor women. 'Toss the Bobbin' was written from the perspective of four of those real women, and although I really didn't think of it at the time, was written by mining the ability to understand and feel the experience of another human from their perspective, that is to empathise. In the way that the novelist must embody her characters to truly evoke any emotion in the reader, the songwriter and the singer must do the same. It's a reincarnation of emotions that you have felt or observed in others. The imagining of pain, joy, loss, love, longing, grief, lust, is integral to the meaningful delivery of a song.

I spend my life with songs. Singing them, learning them, writing them and above all listening to them. I think what I admire most in a singer is the willingness to be vulnerable. To be open to pain as well as joy. For me, it's never how accurately they hit the notes or how well they can control their breath. I really don't care for fancy singing. I'd much rather be moved than impressed. I need to believe the singer. Does the man in the corner of the front bar singing a hundred-year-old song actually care about what that person was going through? Can he feel it for those few moments? Is he really in that autumn day when he saw her first and knew? Does the singer on the stage, with her eyes closed and her brow furrowed really feel the loss of the one she once loved with fond affection? Because if she can't feel it, then I can't. And we will never reach that collective moment as an audience, a group of strangers that allows us to transcend and experience something outside of ourselves, something at another level that somehow connects us all.

A song only survives down through the ages because it resonates, it offers an immediate connection with someone who may have lived in a very different time and place and reminds us that our journeys are not that different after all. Even a century later something still makes the listener hush the pub and say 'Shhh lads, give her a chance'.

I'm thinking of the woman in the front row who takes off her glasses to wipe away the tears that drench her face as the band play 'So Long Marianne'. I'm thinking of the two grown men who throw their arms around each other and venture 'I love you man' as they compose themselves for the encore. I'm thinking of the woman who leans across and clutches the old man's hand as she remembers her mother and knows that they're both thinking of her at that moment. It is empathy that pervades all of these magic moments, and empathy that creates them. From the writing of the song to its delivery, the ability to feel and understand the experience of others is central.

If engaging with art can remind us to do this, and even cultivate within us a greater ability to understand another's feelings and perspective, it can only be beneficial for us as a society. If it contributes in any tiny way to a person's understanding of another, within that there is a real power to change things. There's even the possibility that your friend will think twice before he throws away that remark about the Travellers. Or that they might understand why that child needs asylum in our town. They might consider for one second what might have led to that woman begging on the street. Imagine a night in a country pub where you don't have to search for the words to call out from those around you, even from the mouths of those you love dearly. The casual bigotry, the blatant misogyny, the ubiquitous racism. It'll take more than a few paintings or songs to change this, and more than empathy to eradicate it. But it's surely a good place to start and worth concentrating on, if you ask me.

Empathy in Music Therapy

Rebecca O'Connor

In a recent music therapy session I sat on the floor next to a five-year-old child who'd had a recent car accident, leaving her with complex injuries. She was crying as she lay under the piano in the music therapy room of the hospital whimpering, 'I'm sad', between quiet sobs. In an attempt to reach her through the medium of music, I improvised, gently on the flute in a minor key, aiming to attune to and reflect her sadness, her vocal sounds and breathing patterns. Gradually she calmed and reached out to a nearby xylophone. She began to match my music and took part in a long turn taking, musical conversation, her musical and emotional responses indicated a clear non-verbal understanding, that she had felt heard and understood. Even though I have been practising music therapy for thirty years now, I am always struck by how powerful music is as a therapeutic tool, to connect, share emotions and reach people beyond any language limitations.

Our ability to create and empathetically respond to music is a fundamental part of being human. Music therapy is a profession that utilises this innate ability to respond to music to support people with a range of difficulties and needs. At the National Rehabilitation Hospital (NRH), Dublin I work with children and adults who have had an acquired brain injury, spinal cord injury or limb absence following a traumatic event or illness. In music therapy sessions, clients are invited to use participative music making, familiar music, lyric analysis and song writing to connect and work towards the understanding of a variety of emotions and to support rehabilitation.

Research has shown that music can stimulate all areas of the brain; engaging neural networks that are shared with 'non-musical' cognitive, motor, emotional and language functions. Therefore, it is a unique and powerful therapeutic tool that can be applied through methods and techniques to support recovery, specifically following brain injury. At the NRH music therapy is integrated within a team of nurses, psychologists, occupational therapists, physiotherapists, speech and language therapists and social workers. Music based methods are used in joint sessions where the music becomes the 'glue' that connects the team and the patient.

For example, I recently worked with a speech and language therapist to help a gentleman who had suffered a stroke. His speech was profoundly affected and he had severe difficulty communicating and expressing himself, and it was difficult for others to understand him. I have repeatedly seen that following a brain injury like this, it's the simple things that people really miss; for this gentleman it was to be able to order a pint of Guinness at the pub, the way he would every Friday night before his injury. The empathetic support he needed was for us to understand and help him express what was important to him, so in joint sessions we used a music therapy method called Melodic Intonation Therapy, I wrote a simple song using only the words 'pint of Guinness please', which we sang repeatedly in our sessions. He recorded the song on his phone and was motivated to practise it many times each day with the nurses and his family. On his return from weekend leave, on his last week at the hospital, he and his wife both reported with absolute delight that he had been able to go to his local pub and order a pint of Guinness for himself and his friends.

The use of meaningful familiar songs and analysing the significance of lyrics, is also another powerful tool to help people to express themselves. A young girl I worked with had a spinal cord injury following a car accident, leaving her in a wheelchair. She found it very difficult to express how she was feeling as a result of her traumatic life-changing injuries. When asked how she was feeling, she would just reply that she was 'fine'. In joint sessions with music therapy and psychology we focused on using familiar music to help her find a way to express herself as well as to empathetically connect with and support her emotionally. She chose the song 'I'm a survivor' by Destiny's Child as her personal theme tune and was able to use the song lyrics to work through her experience and constructively express herself in an age appropriate way.

Music can also be used to provide a vehicle for mutual understanding of how others think and feel in group music therapy sessions. In group sessions with young people who, following their brain injuries, have many communication difficulties, music becomes a way in which each group member can connect and also reciprocate and acknowledge each other's feelings. I often see patients who have lost their speech, expressing themselves and developing empathetic connections through music in this way.

Music touches every one of us, no matter who we are. It is a universal language of emotion. By utilising music as a therapeutic tool in music therapy sessions it is possible to empathetically support and connect with people, helping them to reach their potential, express difficult emotions and maximise recovery.

I feel extremely lucky and privileged over many years to have had the opportunity to work with so many clients and team members who have shown me how the powerful language of music can be used to help others to maximise their potential and feel more understood.

Don't Murray, Be Happy!

Cathal Murray

My name is Cathal Worry. I changed it to Murray for show business. For the last five years, I've been at the helm of one of Ireland's longest running late night radio programmes. *Late Date* goes out from 11 p.m. until 2 a.m. seven days a week and I present it from Sunday to Thursday. I consider it a vital part of my job description to empathise with my audience. If I don't consider my listeners and their lives, I'm not doing my job correctly.

Radio listenership is at its highest in the morning and at its lowest at night time. In the morning, the wireless whirs away in the background with news, current affairs, music and zany banter. It's all whatever you're having yourself. It's often background noise while we go about our daily lives; getting ready for work, doing the school run, etc. We mainly listen passively. At night, it's different even though the listening figures are lower. Everyone who's listening is actively listening. People are often alone at home, going to bed with just the radio and my voice for company. It's my duty to deliver a programme that provides a friend if required, or simply the right musical accompaniment for the night.

I feel very lucky to be able to share the music I love with an audience every night. It's all about winding down the day and that's reflected in my selection of music, which is pretty laid back. I often wonder if there is a link between empathy and anxiety. As Ireland went into its first lockdown in March 2020, my anxiety dance card was already full. My wife Siobhán was four months pregnant with our first child, we were trying to buy a house in a difficult property market and my older brother who has an intellectual disability was being treated for lung cancer. I was acutely aware that the rest of the population was probably experiencing similar anxieties with separation from loved ones and forced isolations on the cards. I realised I was in the fortunate position to be able to provide some solace at night in a small way through my job.

People were tuning in looking for a distraction from all the bad and sad news. I made sure to keep mentions of Covid to a minimum. I played the music every night hoping that it made a difference to someone, the way it helped me. Music has the power to make us feel happy or sad or nostalgic and consequently can increase our empathy. Some of the greatest songwriters of all time were empaths. John Prine's song 'Hello in There' really connected with a lot of listeners during this time.

The singer Jonathan Richman tells his girl: 'I got faith in you'. Similarly in Simon and Garfunkel's 'Bridge over Troubled Water', 'if you need a friend I'm sailing right behind'.

Radio provides a real feeling of community – in these days of 'on-demand' with millions of songs ready to stream just a click away there's something about hearing a song that means something to you on the wireless and knowing that someone else is listening, be it in bed, at work, on the road and even scattered around the globe. Radio 1 has a very large global audience made up of Irish residents, expats and a smorgasbord of people with or without an Irish connection who are listening to the radio in their time zone when it's 11 p.m. in Ireland.

I often felt a responsibility during the pandemic to let people know that we are all in this together. Listeners would text, email and tweet messages of hope and defiance – and I was in a privileged position to play songs to reflect those – 'there is a crack in everything that's how the light gets in' (Leonard Cohen), 'All things must pass' (George Harrison), I could fill the rest of the pages of this book with examples.

I hoped the songs helped the listeners – as they helped me. Music is a kind of social glue – the emphatic music from the songwriters mentioned above and so many more made living with this new reality a little bit more bearable – if only for the few minutes they were on the air.

As I write this, my ten-month-old son Joseph is slowly starting to walk and putting all sorts of things he shouldn't into his mouth. My wife and I are both awaiting our second Covid-19 vaccine. My eighty-three-year-old mother left Athlone for the first time since our wedding in December 2019 and came to visit our new house in Dublin and my brother Noel is hanging in there. I'm listening to a song written and released during lockdown by the Irish singer Vyvienne Long called 'A Glass of Laughter'.

> We'll learn to embrace again
> Run the rat race again
> We'll laugh at bad jokes and then
> dance with ol folks again
> We'll cheer when the curtain falls
> Fight back the tears and the wild applause.

This experience will change us, no doubt, hopefully giving us an ability to better understand each other and how fragile we all are. Empathy.

My Essay on Empathy

Tolü Makay

What is empathy?

'The ability to understand and share the feelings of another, from their point of view rather than your own'. A sincere connection, putting yourself in their shoes, acting in that person's best interest.

When asked to write about empathy, I panicked. Self- doubt and overthinking overstayed its visit making me question what I know and if I know enough to be sharing my thoughts. But isn't this an everyday recurring type of issue everyone faces? When I shared this mini fear with a friend, a tip I got was, no matter how many people have probably talked about what you want to talk about, the way you will say it will be your own way. So use your voice, someone will listen. Being listened to and given just that bit of advice, helped calm the storm of thoughts brewing in my mind. It even gave me the boost of confidence I needed. I was listened to, we tried to understand where these doubts were coming from and a solution was provided. I wasn't made to feel like the worries I felt were miniscule. At that moment that's all I needed.

To be empathetic is to actively help in whatever capacity you can. I didn't know having empathy was something that needed to be developed until the day I was attentive in one of my psychology classes. So if empathy isn't innate, it can be taught.

Throughout my years spent on this earth thus far, my idea of why and how people choose to behave has changed continuously. When I was much younger (although taught to be considerate of other people's feelings and how my actions may affect them), whatever didn't fit the idea of what I'd been taught, didn't match the norms of what I saw in my environment or expectations of what a successful person was, I judged.

As I get older, I realised not everyone is operating with the same tools and that privilege plays a huge part making it difficult for some to achieve their goals. You get older again and realise there isn't just one way of solving a problem, so why subscribe to the norm. Going out more and meeting different types of people and collaborating brought about a wider understanding of the multiple ways people live their lives. It made me understand more, listen more, question more, and want to work on being a better human.

The same way something great could happen and change someone's life for the better, is also the same way a terrible moment could change someone's life for the worst in an instant, and sometimes not even a fault of their own.

Vulnerability is a key component. I myself struggle with vulnerability because I need to feel safe with who I share with. To be vulnerable is to share parts of who you are. This can be very daunting. If you haven't yet experienced or understood the importance of vulnerability and what it means to be vulnerable, creating a space of vulnerability for others to speak will be challenging, it can be uncomfortable, given that we live in a society where sharing your feelings isn't rewarded.

I was reading a reddit post about a guy asking whether he was the bad friend in a situation regarding how he handled his friend opening up about their mental health issues. His friend had shared much about their mental health and he became uncomfortable. Instead of listening and trying to understand he told his friend to stop telling him and go seek other help, dismissed him and moved on to another topic. A little empathy in that situation would've been all that's needed. He could have asked, how do you feel right now or is there anything I can do to help, or involve his friend in even trying to figure out the best person he would be comfortable going to.

I think it's also important to touch on social media and how empathy can be practised online. Social media is a lot of people's version of life, their reality and everyday activity. Over the years, we have seen the effects of online bullying and how insensitive posts have ruined people's lives, self esteem, etc. We are a society that bases our status, standard, goals and expectations from social media. We take it seriously. We find love there, soul mates, plan events, find a sense of community, etc. So we should be aware and conscious when online. Empathy doesn't stop and only relate to humans you like, it's being mindful and respectful to every living thing you encounter, including animals and plants. Truly caring for how we treat things around us. We aren't perfect but a bit of empathy will go a long way.

The Light in Somebody Else's Storm

The Very Rev. Lynda Peilow

In my life as a priest, rector and hospital chaplain there have been many hospital visits. It's a demanding role and yet it's also deeply rewarding. As I go from ward to ward, working through my list I never know who or what I will come across. Sometimes I take a deep breath as I knock on the door or call through a curtain. With every visit, I am acutely aware of the vulnerability of the soul in the hospital bed. It's a place where people need the careful care and the company of another human being. Someone who will relate to what they are going through – the loss, the regret, the hidden pain, the unrealised dreams, the sense of helplessness and for some hopelessness. It is a privileged role but one which demands and expects empathy.

The scene can be set in that moment when the phone rings. 'Reverend, it's the ward Sister, we need you to come'. I gather up my keys, my prayer book and I go. As I open the door of the hospital ward, I see a family with tear-stained faces and red rimmed eyes, worn out and exhausted, waiting and watching, hoping and praying, wondering, and wishing. The beeps of the machines working in harmony but playing an unknown tune. That sound becomes very familiar, comforting but intrusive. I make eye contact with everyone so I can communicate any presence not just physically but also emotionally.

I am there to minister, not just to the patient, and the family, but to the hospital staff as well. Everyone is in a space that is far from comfortable, and for some it's life changing. I stand by the bed, let the patient who is slipping in and out of consciousness, know that I am there, place my hand on their forehead and in a calm voice tell them they are surrounded by their family. 'We are all here for you'. In the last few months, I have been part of many scenes like this, listened, prayed, reflected and connected with people in the final hours of this life.

In those moments, there is reverence, there is quiet calm. Amidst the tears there is also often release. As noisy and intrusive as that room may be, it is holding the gathering and uniting each one of us in the experience. This is a sacred space, and there is a way of being and doing that is both necessary and needed, for whatever may follow. As we all unite in saying the Lord's Prayer, voices break and the family hold hands, and then some voices get stronger and louder. Everyone is feeling and reacting differently. In that space, I need to remain present, and yet in order to be present, I am transported into a part of me that feels their pain and anguish.

Some of us step outside into the relative's room. I boil the kettle as the family hold one another, some silent, some sobbing. We sit, we drink tea and then we chat and there are long periods of quiet staring at the mugs, but it's not uncomfortable. The vigil lasts for a few days, and there is safety and sanctuary in that room and hospital ward. Stories flow over the next couple of days, do you remember, if only, what if. They sit, they stretch, there's small talk, they hug, they laugh, they cry, some close their eyes, waken with a jolt, and realise it's not a dream. There is nail biting and handholding.

A loved one who has travelled from overseas might arrive in a panicked exhaustion and falls into the arms of the little group one by one, searching for answers. Seeing my collar, asking if they are too late, I shake my head and I am asked to take them into the ward and so I do, giving them space but letting them know I am there, a hand on their back.

In that place, in this environment we are connected. How we respond and care for one another will ripple out into the future long after the funeral. In fact, a bond grows because of the shared experience and this pain of grief and loss, waiting and watching is felt, shared, understood, held in what has become a sacred space. No one is judged for their tears, their reactions or lack of them, because everyone is coping in their own way. There is patience and a depth of understanding and amidst some members of the little group, a rift might be healed.

It's painful too to be an onlooker when we feel helpless and we cannot take away the suffering of another, but we can stand by. There are no words to utter but there is a silent communication in being present. When a person is slipping into eternity and medical science has done all it can, there remains nothing more than being there, standing by. There is power in the love of being present and it is stronger medicine than we could ever realise. There is a potent therapy in the knowledge that someone cares enough about you to stand by in those hours of need.

And so, it goes for me the hospital bedside, the relatives' room, the chat at the kitchen table, the planning of a funeral, the roadside where someone has collapsed, the telephone, the hospice, the walk on the prom, the eyes that look right into you after a service pleading the need to talk, the silent tears cried by a member of the congregation during a sermon. These people need empathy, not sympathy. They need to connect and to be heard in a non-judgement place.

The world needs brave people who will reach in and out to others, it needs love, compassion, trust, and a space where we can just be, with no judgement, no awkwardness, and no uncomfortable feelings. No matter what is going on in our lives, no matter what emotions are tearing us apart, there is always a part of us that puts on the brave face. Don't let others see, because if they see they might judge us. Perhaps we fear that more than anything else.

Isolation. Hopeless. Helpless. Lonely. Heartbroken. Anxious. Afraid. Misunderstood. Depressing. Alone. Hurting. Healing. Empty. Broken. Distressed. Numb. Shocked. Traumatised. These feelings and emotions are all difficult and challenging parts of the human journey. They impact some lives more severely than others depending on situations and circumstances. All of us need a soft place to land, and be received, as do our feelings and experiences. This can only happen in a non-judgmental environment where there is trust and understanding. Often for us to be able to move forward we may have to circle back where feelings are felt and pain is acknowledged. We all need people who give us the space 'to be' and 'to feel' understood. Empathy is a powerful tool against isolation and dark moments in life of pain, shame, grief, fear and loneliness. It can be transformative and may well be the light in somebody else's storm.

Too Sensitive

Louise O'Neill

When asked what I was like as a child, my mother always pauses, just for a second. She replies with one word – 'different'. Only I can hear the slight hesitation in her voice as she attempts to put a shape on something she could not understand. Then she tells a story, one she thinks will help explain what she means by 'different'. I was five, she says, maybe six, and we are visiting my grandfather in the hospital after he had his hip replaced. I sit on his bed, stealing pink iced caramels. The nurse asks me if I would like to be a nurse when I am grown up. According to my mother, I stare at her and ask, 'why would I be a nurse and not a doctor?' And then, popping another sweet in my mouth, I say, 'anyway. I'm not going to be either. I'm going to be an actress.' Apart from a very brief period of wanting to be a nun (a prerequisite for a Catholic childhood, I think), that was all I ever wanted. I dreamt of a life on the stage, an eager audience before me. I was going to brand my name on the seas of this planet until every last person knew who I was.

I often wonder what my childhood self would think of me now. How my thirty-six-year-old self craves solitude rather than applause, thrives on the plodding routine of going to my desk at the same time every day and seeing what magic I can create on the blank page before me. And even now, if there was to be a third act to my career, I cannot imagine it will involve the theatre. Rather, I am drawn to psychology. I picture myself as something close to what a dear friend and I describe as a Cashmere Therapist; an older woman with chic grey hair and draped in scarves, scribbling session notes in her monogrammed leather notebook. But when I look at these three careers – acting, writing, therapy – the other lives I could be living in a parallel universe to this one, I can see the common thread that weaves through them all. It is the desire to examine the human condition, to walk in another's shoes and hear their heart beat as your own. To understand why people behave the way that they do. To understand them. Empathy, I suppose you could call it.

And yet for such a long time, I tried to fight my empathetic tendencies. It was all-too easy for me to sink into the pain of another, to internalise their experience as my own. I would come home from school distraught because another student had been reprimanded by the teacher, and then again when another child's grandparent had died. I had an affliction, you see, I could not distinguish between my classmate's suffering and my own. Having cried to my mother, she would sigh that I needed a tougher skin, I was too sensitive. Looking back, it's obvious that she was worried and trying to protect me in the best way she could. She knew the world would be unforgiving if I remained that porous and what I needed in order to be happy was to establish appropriate boundaries, although she didn't have the language to articulate it in that way. But it wasn't until my uncle died that my sensitivity became a problem.

I am fourteen. My sister and I retrying on bridesmaid dresses, admiring ourselves in the mirror when the phone rang. Then my mother's voice. 'Just tell me,' she says. 'Is he dead?' Turning around to stare at her. 'Is it Dad?' I ask. 'No,' she replies. 'It's Michael. There's been an accident.' We drive to my grandparents' farmhouse, my mother's knuckles white as she grips the steering wheel. When we pull up outside, I can hear the wailing already, and then it is chaos – bodies everywhere and my grandfather sobbing like a child and my grandmother, sitting so still, her hands clasped in her lap. I go to her, like I always did, looking for comfort, for love, and she stares up at me and says, 'I'll have to get my hair done, I suppose'.

My uncle was thirty and when someone dies that young, it destabilises everything you take for granted about life. Suddenly, the world seems unsafe, precarious; anyone can be taken from you at any moment. Over those next few days, I felt as if I was in a nightmare I could not wake up from. Falling, falling, falling, waiting for the concrete to meet me. Watching his fiancée, only twenty-six herself, sink to her knees, keening. I remember that I was unable to stop crying, I was verging on hysterical – I couldn't tell the line between where my grief ended and the terror began, the fear that this was only the beginning and that everyone I loved would be taken from me, one by one. A family member took me aside and informed me that my 'dramatics' couldn't continue. That if I didn't get my act together, they would stop me from going to the funeral or they would give me a sedative to shut me up. It strikes me now as an unbearably cruel thing to say to a fourteen-year-old girl but at the time, I accepted this as fair. I stopped crying that day and it would be almost a decade before I cried again. I completely shut down, turning to an eating disorder to numb out any painful emotions. I didn't feel sad anymore but I wasn't particularly happy either. I didn't feel anything at all.

I kept acting for a while after that but I had lost the heart for it. By the time I left for university, I had packed away my dreams of studying theatre under the bed, like it was a doll I no longer had any use for, and instead chose English Studies. It's more sensible, I said, but I wonder if acting simply felt too dangerous. A part of me knew I would have to tap into those raw emotions in order to be convincing on stage and I thought if I did that, I might die. I don't think it's any coincidence that when I had a breakthrough in my recovery, when I finally broke down in the therapy room and wept, that it felt like something had shifted when it came to my creativity too, and I yearned to make art again.

Here's the thing – if you can't have empathy for yourself, then it's extraordinarily difficult to have empathy for other people. It's difficult to find the space to hold their pain when you're busy trying to suppress your own. And we need empathy, now more than ever before. It is what makes us human. It's what connects us to one another. When we wake in the middle of the night, our bleakest fears casting shadows on the walls, empathy is what reminds us that we are not alone, we have never been alone. There have been people before us who experienced this – this heartbreak, this grief, this love, this joy – and there will be people after us who will do the same. We are more alike than we are different, I suppose. And so now, as I go about my day, I look for moments to express empathy. To look at another and say – I see you, I understand you.

Isn't that what we all want?

To be seen.

To be understood.

Empathy Checkpoint

Martina Venneman

It's almost midnight and the phone rings in the garda station. When we answer the phone, the caller sounds unsure and at the same time in a rush to tell us a story about their life. We haven't spoken before and we have two immediate questions for them. Are they safe right now or in danger? They are safe, their children are asleep in bed. What's their name and phone number so that we can contact them, if they are cut off? We make a note of their details. They explain to us about the things they have been experiencing at home recently and how their spouse's behaviour towards them and their children is upsetting them. We listen as they tell us about incident after incident and apologise for the jumbled up way they're presenting the details. We believe their story to be legitimate and accept their version of events in good faith. Our empathy has kicked in: we understand the caller needs space to tell their story, and that it has been a big deal for them to pluck up the courage to make contact with the local garda station.

We recognise the caller is reporting domestic abuse and we are familiar with the law that makes it a crime. We might interrupt them to tell them about the law relating to domestic violence and what they can generally expect from the legal system. This is legitimate and practical information, but it could result in 0the caller feeling overwhelmed by what we're telling them they should do. They might end the call early, and the abuse they are experiencing at home is likely to continue and also become progressively worse for them. Instead, we listen to their story and we hear that they feel trapped, confused and helpless and that they are desperate to protect their children from this. Why is this happening to them? they wonder.

When we see the situation from the caller's point of view, we can use our judgement and experience to advise them about the options they have right now. Based on what they've told us, we can explain the actions we will take and make suggestions for things that they might consider doing. Acknowledging the caller's fear is an important part of our role, understanding and respecting that they might feel reluctant when we ask them to take a number of difficult steps. Things like telling a friend or relative about the abuse for example, or to consider leaving the family home, arranging for their children to be looked after by a friend or relative, or making contact with domestic violence services. We are using empathy as the key to understanding their feelings and emotions, and also how much they are willing to take on at this time. This guides us in providing the appropriate response to the caller, to support them as much as we can to tackle the domestic abuse and the effect it is having on their lives and that of their children. Our work protocols guarantee that the caller will receive the information and help they require, but it is the tool of empathy that allows us to connect with the victim and to tailor our intervention based on what they've told us about their individual situation. When we offer support and guidance beyond generic procedures and practices, we are even more likely to achieve a positive outcome for the caller and their children.

Later that day our unit is assigned to police a street protest. Some of the people protesting are pushing their way forward and are shouting loudly in our faces as we get in the way of where they want to go. We are familiar with people acting angrily toward us and taunting us, making it clear to us that they are frustrated or unhappy with our presence. This can happen in a number of different situations, for example when stopping motorists at checkpoints, calling to people's homes to help with resolving family disputes and conflicts with neighbours, or patrolling on a street late at night. In all cases where people are agitated and unwilling to engage, it is not helpful to take it personally, or react impulsively and get caught up in a lengthy exchange of views and opinions, explaining our role and our position. As well as having very little positive effect, individual confrontations also diminish our command of the situation and our effectiveness as a unit. Having one member engaged in a heated argument with one of the people protesting becomes the main focus, and this disrupts the unity and strength of our team as a whole, distracting from our wider task of safely policing the protest.

Although it is often very challenging, it is an important skill to be able to respect and acknowledge the views of the people protesting. It does not mean that we fully – or even partially – agree with their cause or the manner in which they are promoting their message. However, this skill is essential to looking after everybody's safety and to work together and engage with the people protesting, to minimise chaos and maintain order in the vicinity. It's very likely that the issue of the protest will influence our reaction in one way or another, but even a more detached form of empathy will help us to police this situation peacefully. When fear, frustration and rage are recognised and acknowledged, it is less likely to lead to confrontation and misunderstanding, or escalate to conflict and violence. At the same time, empathy opens the door to the possibility of co-operation and allows for a more positive and peaceable result.

At the end of the shift when we are finished work, we

might reflect on what the day has brought. Our tendency will probably be to be critical of ourselves and remember the things that didn't go perfectly. While we are evaluating our actions and reactions, we use empathy to recognise our own feelings and regrets without any inner judgement or blame. Empathy towards ourselves is a type of self-compassion or kindness that allows us to understand our reasons for doing what we did, even when we did not achieve the success we wanted. By using empathy, it steers us away from shame, guilt and self-hatred, and more in the direction of respect, care and compassion for ourselves, valuing our own efforts and contributions. Practising self-compassion in this way gives us an opportunity to tune in to what we really want, and the way we are striving to make positive, helpful and effective contributions in the situations we encounter. Armed with this powerful tool of empathy, and with the knowledge and insight it gives us about ourselves and others, we are ready to make a fresh start and face the challenges and responsibilities of our next workday.

Showing Empathy to Youth

Gary Nugent

When I set out thinking about my experiences of empathy I thought that it would be easy for me, I am a youth worker, surely that makes me a professional empath? And it's true I have many examples for times where I showed empathy to young people and families, but then I began to explore why and where my empathy had come from. I wondered why I have chosen a career that demands so much empathy, and so I spent some time looking back at people that had showed me empathy and the experiences that had led me to where I am today.

Growing up in rural Ireland I found it difficult to find my place, not being into sports and struggling with my identity. It was when I joined my local youth club that I found a place where I felt I could be myself and show my strengths. While being part of Foróige, I had the opportunity to join their national youth reference panel, in the world of young people in Foróige this was a pretty big deal. I remember being collected in my local town by a youth worker called Gerry who was driving a Foróige bus to the reference panel in Dublin, collecting young people between Galway and Dublin along the way. Getting onto that bus, I didn't know the impact that this one weekend would have on me. Being in a bubble of positivity and young people with the same interests was so incredible, however I really hadn't prepared myself for the weekend to end. Getting on the bus home with my new-found friends was great, keeping the weekend going a little longer.

When we reached the town where I was due to depart, I

was inconsolable to have to say goodbye to the people and the feeling of belonging that I had found. Gerry the youth worker was so kind and saw how difficult that I was finding it. He turned off the bus and said to us all 'sure we might take a break here for a few minutes and get some chips'. This had not been his plan and was done solely to allow me a little extra time to deal with what I thought was my world ending. This small bit of extra time really meant a lot to me and the empathy that he showed to me made the situation so much easier. I often think about how he had spent the full weekend working, away from his own children and wife but was still willing to give even more to help out a kid be had only met two days previous.

Fast forward about fifteen years and I have been a youth worker for nearly ten years. I recently got and email from a young person that I had worked with during a youth leadership event. This is a five-day event with young people from all over Ireland and different parts of the world. The young person was contacting me to ask if I could support them in completing their portfolio. Having facilitated the programme to hundreds of young people I was unsure who this specific young person was, so I asked him to give me some further details. His response was one that I hadn't expected. He replied 'This is kind of embarrassing but you may remember that you bought me a shirt from Dunnes for the gala (which I still appreciate thank you).' Instantly I recall the young person and the occasion. I remember that the young person felt that they could not attend the gala dinner, the highlight of the week, just because they didn't have a shirt to wear. I remember thinking I could just tell the young person that it doesn't matter what you wear and they could just wear whatever they had. However, I knew how it felt to feel as if you didn't fit in and if something as simple as a shirt could ease the young person's worries and let them really enjoy their night then it was a very small cost for a great reward. It's amazing that I left the next day and never thought about it again, but three years later that young person remembered, and it still meant a lot to them. I wondered how he still remembered it and then I thought about how fifteen years later every time I see Gerry the youth worker from the bus I always remember how kind he had been and the impact he made on me.

When I first started on this piece I was fully sure that I would have some extravagant example of how I had saved the world with a grand display of empathy, however it appears that on that front I have not been successful. As I went through the examples, it appeared that none actually made me recall how I felt due to the experience and how it has impacted on the way I show empathy to others. When I think about the way I left on that cold February Sunday evening in a rural midland town I can still remember how Gerry's single action made me feel. I think about my actions with the young person at leadership and how without me even knowing, they had been shaped so many years previous by one simple empathic gesture.

A Traveller's Perspective

Martin McDonagh

As a traveller and a youth worker with Foróige I am very aware of the presence and importance of empathy not just for all youth but for their families and communities. Within the context of the traveller community, culture there is a strong automatic tradition of empathy not least in the context of automatically helping each other in times of need. For example, with the occurrence of the death of a family member, the travelling community automatically 'chips in' by contributing some money towards the costs of the funeral. So the burden does not lie solely with the family, but the community operates a very discrete donation process that kicks in automatically when needed in the immediate aftermath of the person passing away. I see this as a great example of 'automatic empathy in action'. Very often when the settled community view what is seen as an extravagant funeral, false assumption as to how that is paid for may follow, but in fact it is by a large set of small donations from the kindness of fellow neighbours and extended family that the costs are covered. If it were the case that there was a surplus of money when all the funeral costs were covered rather than refund anyone their donation the money leftover would automatically be left with grieving family towards the cost of headstone for the grave.

Empathy was also part of everyday living for me growing up. I come from a family where the role of grandparents as role models and as providers of support to children and grand-children was a key aspect of our regular routine. Not least, I have memories of a grandmother who was so kind when making tea for her family would make enough tea for the many neighbours living nearby.

Whereas this tradition of compassion still exists, I have seen many changes in traveller lifestyles over the years and have some concern that this level of traditional caring amongst the traveller community is changing and not for the good. Just as families in the settled community face issues such as alcohol abuse, domestic violence or gambling, these also are the very same problems for traveller families. Just as there are brilliant role models within both communities there are also those who suffer and struggle – being a traveller or being settled it is all the same in this regard.

One of the unique aspects of giving support for those in need is the importance of doing so in a way that does not belittle the person in need of help – otherwise it is no longer an act of empathy. Given the tight margins between the ages of children and grandchildren in traveller families, where possible support with providing clothing or food to all in need can be accommodated 'under cover'.

Working as a youth worker in the community and regardless of whether I am working with a traveller or settled young person (which is never an issue for me), the key ingredient is that the young person is valued and treated with pure respect, and you can show this best in the way that you deliver help. It is important that the other person realises that needing help is not his/her fault and that bad and sad things can happen to any of us. I have a particular memory of working with a young traveller youth with his trousers that were ripped up to his knee and in very bad condition – it reminded me of my own youth and what I experienced – I may not have walked in his shoes, but I wore those trousers for sure!!!

Rather than act with pure pity which is not a good option, we engaged the young person in a local football club and on route to training made sure he 'mucked up his trousers even more'. This meant that after practice he would have to shower and as per normal for anyone in that position we gave him replacement trousers from our stock for this regular occurrence – and washed his torn trousers to bring home with him as well. The important thing is that empathy is best served if the person is not singled out and it is just a natural process.

Overall if I think about empathy as a traveller and working with the settled community, I have learned to see it from both sides and I have seen and witnessed the total racism and discrimination that many travellers face daily.

That aside, I have learned the key thing is not to judge people based on them being a traveller or settled. Judge them as the person they are. Just as we need empathy for all older people (traveller and settled), a tradition that is to some extent not as strong as perhaps it was, we need to show empathy by enjoying older people, respecting them and supporting them and certainly not to label them because of their age.

It is a dangerous path to be on if we lose respect and empathy for others. Who do you turn to if you have a bad time? Who do you feel you can talk to? We need to see the other person as the other person not the traveller or not the settled. We are not born with racism, we must learn it. For me it is all about doing to others what you would like them to do with and for you. It may be surprising to say this, but humour is part of empathy and done properly, and not with discrimination, is a great form of communication. Ultimately I want those I work with to see me Martin as a good person and a good youth worker. After over twenty years in this work, I have learned the best result I can get is if those I work with see me as a sound person not just as a traveller or a youth worker. I have learned that with empathy, if I give respect I always get it back.

Empathy through Food

Michelle Darmody

When eating and cooking together a tacit language emerges. Even if we do not share the same native language we can communicate through food, break bread together, after all the word companion means 'with bread', its origins can be traced back to – com ('with') and panis ('bread'). Bread, as with many foods, has long been associated with sharing, nurturing and friendship. Food binds us together and is essential for life, both physical and social. The recent inability to touch, or hug, or to share bread together due to COVID-19 has highlighted, with an ever brighter intensity, the importance of these human connections. Interactions once tactile and exuberant are now fraught and fragile.

Food is a part of everyone's life, but I seem to have embroiled myself with it in many ways: I have earned my living through food, I avidly read novels or research based on food and I passionately believe that it can be used as a tool for positive change. When food is seen as a commodity, and only that, it becomes devoid of many of the facets that nourish us and the world around us; respect for the biodiversity of our land and sea is lost

To encourage empathy through food we can of course sit and eat together but it stretches further, it stretches into the fields and into the soil beneath those fields. We need to show empathy for those who till the land, and care for the living, breathing soil that provides our nourishment. The complicated food system we have developed for ourselves has so many tendrils it is hard to trace them back to the farm or to the soil. In the factory, we often see poor conditions and even poorer practices where food is removed from nature and people are left with no choice but to work in poorly paid positions, often separated from those they love.

With deforestation, we can see the destruction of habitats and the damage that is so devastating it has moved the world into a new epoch. There are alternatives ways of working in harmony with the earth as well as its people.

When running from violence and unrest many people shed all of their belongings on the journey, arriving to a new place with little or nothing. One thing that does cross borders is recipes. The taste of home can be a comfort in dark times and food often provides people with a new start in a new land. Setting up a food project called Our Table taught me this. I had the pleasure of cooking with people from many different countries and most had battled adversity to get to Irish shores. The project aimed to highlight the inhumanity of the fact that people living in Direct Provision were not allowed to cook for themselves. Many people are trapped in the system for years on end and the lack of cooking and choosing what food to eat impacts their family life, and their physical and mental well-being.

Our Table was set up in conjunction with Ellie Kisyombe, who came to Ireland seeking political asylum and ended up in Direct Provision for nine years. The stifling system wears people down in many ways but being fed low cost, processed food every day, three times a day, with no end in sight is one particularly cruel aspect. At the beginning of Our Table, we simply provided a kitchen and boxes of ingredients, and people came from the Direct Provision centres and we cooked together. It was extremely emotive, we ate, we cried, we listened to each other's stories, all the time making delicious food. I learned how to create a very good pot of jollof rice, to make bajilé, which are like falafel made with beans, and to bake intricate Syrian pastries. After a few such cooking days, there was talk of doing a more public facing event, one that brought our conversation into the public domain. The Project Arts Centre in Temple Bar allowed us to use their large theatre space and we set up a three-day café, people could either eat for free or leave a donation. We were overwhelmed by the support. I realised that many people in the wider community wanted to show solidarity and empathy with those in Direct Provision but had no outlet to do so. We provided that outlet for many and at the same time garnered support from the media. Ellie still runs Our Table and it still has shared cooking at its core.

In a brighter tomorrow we could begin to create all food with care, as if it were to be shared with those we love, making and breaking bread with empathy at its heart.

Reflections on Empathy and Sport

Eamonn O'Shea

Empathy is not the first thing that comes to mind when trying to build the identikit of the ideal inter-county hurling manager, which I once was for a short period of three years. The golden rule of competitive sport is to win – the narrative for high level elite competition is rooted in combat, battle, attrition and war. Don't look backwards or sideways, make sure your sword is sharp and your shield is strong, and, above all, leave any concern for your opponent at home. It's hard for empathy to surface, let alone flourish in such a world. 'Them's the rules and you live or die by them', as the saying goes. But, is that always true and is there another way of looking at empathy in sport?

This reflection is rooted at the end of my time as manager of the Tipperary senior hurling team in 2015 when one of my friends (it is true that there are less of them after a loss!), in an effort to console me on losing my last match in charge of the county, an All Ireland semi-final against Galway, casually remarked that 'I probably had too much empathy to be a really successful manager'. Leaving aside that she was showing little empathy herself at this time, I was too annoyed at losing and exhausted from the experience to understand, let alone contest, this judgement. Although I did wonder at the time what journalists interviewing me after the game might have made of it, if, in explanation of the loss I said, 'just put it down to empathy – we simply had too much of it today. So much so, that we spent the day appreciating the feelings of the other team rather than doing anything ourselves'. But the accusation of 'too much empathy' lingered, leading me to contemplate whether excessive (or indeed any) empathy is good or bad in sport?

The Chambers Dictionary tells us that empathy is 'the power of entering into another's personality and imaginatively experiencing his or her experiences'. If I do have too much empathy, I have spent a lot of my life hiding it in relation to sport – just like yourself before you get all self-righteous about it. I have time only for my experiences – my feelings when my team wins and lose matters most.

Opponents and other teams hold little or no interest for me, except as adversaries. I dislike teams easily, mainly on the basis that they are not from where I'm from. The latter being one of the best descriptions ever in explaining GAA culture in Ireland.

When my team wins, I spend zero seconds wondering how the opposition feel about losing or what can be done to ease their pain. The Swedish philosophers Abba called it correctly – the winner takes it all: the loser's standing small. That may explain why I have spent a lot of my time in recent years unsuccessfully trying to devise plans to break down Limerick's impressive and winning way of playing the game of hurling (a plan for the whole game rather than just half the game in case you are a Tipp fan reading this!). I do not spend my time wondering how the champions feel about being so good at the moment or how thrilled I am that they are the current standard-bearers of the game. To give you a flavour of my mood in August 2021, I bought a ticket for the All-Ireland hurling final but just could not bring myself to go to the match, deciding instead to cycle around the streets of Dublin, thinking about anything else but the game. No sign of empathy that day for sure.

But is an unwillingness to bear witness to your rivals'

triumph evidence of an absence of empathy? In the cold light of day, it sounds and feels more like envy rather than empathy or the lack of it. Back to Chambers again, where empathy is also described as 'the power of entering into the feeling or spirit of something (especially a work of art) and so appreciating it fully'. Now that is a definition I can get behind – hurling as art that can only be understood through a creative lens. In truth, I understand only too well when rivals are better. For example, to witness the genius of hurling artists like Tony Kelly and Cian Lynch is liberating and debilitating in equal measure. The latter because you know the consequences for your team; but mainly liberating because you know you are witnessing something joyful and beautiful. For a brief period, you are allowed access to a metaphysical world where the Gods mingle and aesthetics prevail; where to be present for a brief interlude is a gift for those of us close to the hurling action.

But equally perhaps, the pursuit and appreciation of empathy comes from the realisation that aesthetics are not confined to the world of the god's, making it important that we search for it in our everyday ordinary lives. Empathy can help us find extraordinary beauty in ordinary places. The ability to see the lives of others, their successes and failures, through their actual experiences is an important trait in all of us. It is what makes us human. But it takes time and practice, just like the pursuit of sporting excellence. A crucial first step in developing empathy, seeing lives for what they are, is getting rid of judgement on the experiences of others. Instead of judgement, better to walk in the shoes of others sometimes and experience their joy, sadness and everything in-between, it may help us understand the ups and downs of our own journeys.

As a manager and a coach I have delivered messages to young talented athletes which have, at the very least, disrupted their dreams – that they may have progressed as far as they can go in their chosen sport at this time; a question mark for some, a full stop for others. I have often been as devastated in delivering that verdict and they have been in receiving it, knowing that I too was given the same message many times in my own life, and not just in sport. But empathy gives you the confidence to communicate the truth to them that disappointment in one area of life need not diminish the self; that personhood is resilient and strong if nurtured well and supported consistently. If anything, disappointment provides opportunities for people to recalibrate and reimagine a different future where potential and talent continues to be activated, remodelled and realised in many different and beautiful forms. There is never just one life – we live multiple lives across our lifetime.

It should not, of course, be difficult to have empathy with failure in sport, because it happens so often. Managers, coaches and players lose more than they win, so it's not hard to know what others are feeling in such circumstances. Partisan support for your team is good, but you can also seek to interrogate and understand individual success and failure, through appreciating fully the experiences of others. Doing so might help reduce the debilitating tendency in sport nowadays to belittle and demonise losers. Maybe respect initiatives should be complemented by empathy awareness to allow us to recognise the 'other' as ourselves in another coat.

If we want support when we need it most ourselves, it's helpful to think about others and what they might be experiencing in good times and bad. After all, it is mainly through reciprocity and mutual understanding that we make sense of the world. If that is the case, then let's have more empathy, not less, in all aspects of our lives, especially in sport.

Stepping in the Stirrups of Others

Rachael Blackmore

I grew up on a farm and have always loved animals particularly horses. I started riding from the age of three and I am still riding however, now it's my job, my career, although being a professional jockey doesn't feel like a job! I have been very fortune to experience some fantastic days in racing, but this did not occur in an instant, and has spanned two very differing pathways. Over time and with successes and disappointments, I have moved from being unknown and not particularly flourishing to more recent heights of recognition and success. Without realising it one personal 'side benefit' of this two-track career history has enabled me to rediscover and reflect on my own feelings on the importance of acts of friendships from, and empathy towards, other jockeys as well as the obvious need for my on-going care and understanding in working with horses, regardless of their differing capabilities.

During the first half of my riding career things were very slow to get going, I was gaining valuable experience but not with the success I wanted. I rode in many races on horses that were not particularly fancied by the betting public at lower status races. This memory is a far cry from more recent successful years with my now being in the very envious position of having a pick of top grade one horses to ride in Cheltenham or other prestigious festivals. In the first few years there were many occasions where I was often left with a craving for success, wanting to make riding winners a regular thing to emanate the success of other jockeys. And, although things are better now for me, I have not forgotten how quickly things can change in racing and how it feels when things are not going your way.

Subconsciously as I've gone through my career as a jockey, I've learned and improved my empathy for and consideration towards others I work with. Where as I now have the great position of getting on these unbelievable talented horses and participating in the most prestigious races, I can still see and feel how it must be for many of my fellow jockeys who are struggling in a very competitive and demanding profession. As jockeys, we are all aware of how quickly things can change and as the saying goes 'you are only as good as your last winner'.

Horseracing is a very competitive and sometimes unforgiving sport, and as a professional jockey I see it from both sides, I'm still on both sides, you ride a winner in the first race everyone is happy and then go out in the second race and are unseated at the last ten lengths clear of everyone else. Your state of mind can change in an instant.

It has been said that experiencing success (joy) and failure (disappointment) through participating in sport mirrors and reflects life. I think this is true and I can see how winning and losing in some ways helps us to learn and cope, although it doesn't make losing any easier! Given the very tight margins of success or failure in racing – sometimes down to 'a nose' – this may be particularly true.

Empathy isn't Black and White

Joanne O'Riordan

So, what does empathy mean to me? Empathy isn't black and white. It isn't a word with a simple definition or something you can pinpoint. I've worked with psychologists before, particularly sports psychologists, given my work in sport, and they always told me to help athletes deal with feelings and thoughts. They would ask the athletes to put a colour or a shape on that feeling.

Empathy as a colour would definitely be a shade of blue, given how we usually associate it with understanding sadness or tragedy, or how we associate it with gut-wrenching nausea we feel when we see a loved one hurt or upset. We definitely can relate to a loved one feeling pain or suffering.

One story that stands out in my mind where empathy was certainly lacking was when I was a baby. I was born without limbs with a rare condition called Total-Amelia, or *Tetra Amelia* if you want to go full Latin. There are only seven other people in the world living with this condition.

My parents and four older siblings did not know I would be born the way I am until the thirty-week routine scan. The nurse called in the doctor, and the doctor just said what he had to say and walked out. It's probably not something you'd learn in the handbook for empathy.

After I was born, doctors told my parents that despite being healthy even without limbs, they should go to the graveyard, pick a plot of ground and basically prepare for the worst. My parents did just that. Spoiler alert: I'm still here.

I went for the hospital check-up all babies are obliged to

do. The doctor did a routine assessment, and once again, I was reasonably healthy despite having no limbs. But, the doctor had an entirely different view.

As my mother was changing me and putting me back together, he asked her, what do you do with a doll that loses a hand. Confused and taken by surprise, my mother said she had no clue. The doctor said the doll will continue to lose limbs, and by that stage, you should just put the broken doll into a cupboard and forget about it, move on with your life and pretend it never happened.

The metaphorical doll was me, and the metaphorical cupboard was an institution so I could be forgotten about while everyone moved on with their lives. It's disgusting to think about, and probably reading that story, you might feel that gut-wrenching nausea I described earlier.

This is how people with disabilities were treated and still are treated in different countries around the world. Even in Ireland, the limited services that are busting at the seams due to overload and underfunding are pitting kids with disabilities and their families against each other to see who needs the services more.

Don't worry, this story has an upside and a to be continued happy ending. I'm living what I assume is my best life, surrounded by people who love and adore me. In my mother's mind, that's pushing me to be my best self. In my siblings' eyes, that's wrestling me, accidentally knocking out my two front teeth mid-Batista-bomb, or in their words, instilling a toughness into me, I'd need in later years. In my dad's eyes, it's driving me around the country to football matches for our weekend bonding session … others call it my job as a sportswriter.

I've successfully campaigned for disability rights, spoke to the United Nations twice regarding technology for people with disabilities, had a documentary made on my life which has been seen by fifteen million people worldwide. I'm hoping to be a successful sports journalist and, hopefully, broadcaster. You don't see many people without limbs doing that!

And that's down to the empathy other strangers, family members and friends have shown me. Tina Stark, a girl twelve years older than me, born the same as me, did not know my family. Yet she and her adopted family in the UK let my family come over and hang out with them in their house for a week so I could see Tina living her best life. I learned everything I can do today from Tina, including eating, drinking, swimming, college life and even where not to get tattoos.

Looking at my list of achievements and things I enjoy doing, I realised that the very reason I can do these things is because I can feel for other people. When injustice rears its ugly head, I can relate, understand and empathise. But I also have a determination in me unlike any other.

It was that sheer desire to never stop, that relentlessness to change things until they were perfect, and that same attitude to do it myself when I felt that others wouldn't pull their weight.

I think it's important to strive for empathy even when it's challenging. Empathy can be as intense and heavy as having an emotional reaction to someone else's tragedy or as simple as putting your phone away at the dinner table to give everyone your full attention. In today's crazy political and social climate, we need to educate ourselves and show empathy boldly, without any hesitation or fear. It's essential to speak up and out when something matters to us and ask others to show empathy towards specific topics or people.

Telling stories that touch people who you may not know emotionally is what embodies humanity. A more empathetic world, in my view, means a more understanding world. An empathetic environment is more inclusive, selfless and peaceful.

Nursing – in the Blink of an Eye

Marie Lohan

Twelve hours ahead! Walking through the doors of your department, hoping and praying that today will be better than yesterday. Yes! There are days that are better than others – in every job. Some days will make you wonder why you ever picked this as your career, but there are days and in just one brief moment it will justify why you became a nurse.

Nursing for years has been branded a profession. A nurse needs to be kind, caring, have a good sense of humour, be a good communicator and above all have empathy for their patient's. Empathy is something that is in us all as humans, some show it and some don't. As a nurse, you will always try to understand your patient, support them and do what is right for them. We try to remove any pain, anxiety fear and worry where possible during times of ill health. It may not always be possible we will always try our best.

There are always two sides – to look after the patients and their families. During this unforeseen pandemic hundreds of families in our hospital went through all sorts of emotions – fear, anxiety, panic, worry frustration and the unknown which can be the biggest fear of all for patients. It is so important to empathise with your patients to gain their trust. It will improve your communication and strengthen the nurse-patient relationship.

Been a nurse doesn't just mean we administer medications or that we tend the patients activities of daily living. It's much more. As a nurse, we strive to be the best advocate we possibly can be for our patients while also providing comfort and support to them and their families.

I chose to be a nurse because of my granny. She was the most thoughtful, loving, kind, caring and fair women who looked after me during my schooldays while my parents were gone to work. She taught me to appreciate the simple things in life and that the note in your head was much more valuable than the note in your pocket. I've always thought of that as I've grown up.

Fast forward to today. I have been an Emergency Department nurse for the past twelve years. It is challenging ninety-nine per cent of the time to say the least, but everyday I'm grounded and thankful by the fact that it's not me or any of my family members lying on one of those trollies because when we get up in the morning there's not one of us that knows where we'll be in the evening.

I remember when I started working in the Emergency Department as a qualified registered nurse. I was nineteen days a new nurse, emotionally charged awaiting the hundreds of situations that I could be faced with. The department was pre-alerted to a cardiac arrest that was coming in – a cardiac arrest is the abrupt loss of heart function, breathing and consciousness. I was in awe of how skilled the more senior nurses were at their roles and setting up equipment. I will never forget, as long as I live, the fear I had in me. The patient was forty-seven-years old and had a sudden collapse at home. The patient subsequently passed away. I had never met this person or knew anything about them, but the sadness I felt was awful. I will never forget their mother and siblings as they came into see their loved one laid out. I nearly felt that I was equally as upset as them. I couldn't stop the tears as they filled my eyes, trying my best to hold them back as this was their loved one and not mine.

There's not a day that goes by that some little thing doesn't grip you as a nurse and clutches at those heart-strings but that's only normal. I think the day that feelings like that begin to disappear it's time to hang up the boots! Your health is most definitely your wealth.

Empathy from My Mother

Seán Campbell

My mother, Kathleen Campbell, was the most empathetic person I have ever known. Any empathy I have, or have ever shown, was learned from her. She was born at the younger end of a family of twelve and her role as a carer to her younger siblings and older working brothers meant that schooling was an occasional distraction and, as it was delivered through the medium of Irish, an irrelevant chore.

Mammy tried to see the good and the best in everyone. Really tried. To her, everyone had redeeming characteristics, unseen motives and intentions behind their actions. I watched her apply that faith in humanity at a time when the rest of us struggled so much to see past the atrocities on our island. She raised me in a border town at the height of the Troubles. Somehow, through that, she never held hate but tried to avoid judgement to anybody involved. That was God's job. With that, she felt every death, be it British or Irish, Republican or Loyalist, and she cried at every one of them. They were some mother's son.

One of my earliest memories is of the tragic passing of a neighbour's child, struck down by a car. What I remember from that event isn't just the shock or the pain, but the ability of my mother to step immediately into the skin of the bereaved parent. Letting go of graces, my mother went straight to the neighbour's home and got down on her hands and knees, scrubbing a house that wasn't hers clean, for at the time, what your neighbours thought about your home truly mattered –

and no grieving mother should have to think about cleaning. This was empathy in action. My mother did what she could to help, thinking about what she would need if she was in the situation, and tried to lift the burden of another in any way she could.

Her empathy was unsophisticated, in the most beautiful way. She didn't need to philosophise over it, define it, or have it acknowledged. She could just feel how others felt and show kindness in the face of it and accept others at their best. What a wonderful perspective to have on the world.

To many of us, empathy is something we will build throughout our lives. We'll take pieces of it from that which has been shown to us, build it over experiences where we've struggled or watched the struggles of others. For the rare few, it is an innate expression of goodness. It's part of how their mind perceives the world. For Mammy, it was always part of her, intertwined with her Catholic beliefs. And I was privileged to learn it from her, to build it within myself from the path she role modelled.

I didn't know I was learning empathy as I watched her. I was yet to understand that empathy can be taught, learned, practised, mastered and even measured. This revelation came over two decades into my career with Foróige, when an evaluation of the Leadership for Life Programme – which aimed to teach young people leadership skills such as communication and critical thinking – revealed that young people showed statistically significant increases in empathy on completion of the programme. What an incredible insight to know that the best characteristic of humanity is something we can all possess. For those of us who aren't natural carers, we can learn to become this. Knowing this has given me a sense of responsibility. There is no excuse for not exercising empathy. If you don't have it, build it.

This increase in empathy amongst the young graduates of the Leadership for Life Programme was an unintended outcome. Foróige now teaches empathy by design, in programmes built specifically to target this skill and nurture it. I think of how the world would be if all our young people had the opportunity to have this nurtured within them, to see the world just a little bit through the perspective my mother did.

Increased empathy would counteract the anonymity felt on social media, forcing everyone to feel for the real person behind the comments they post, and I'm confident would reduce cyber-bullying. Understanding how our actions have consequences on others and genuinely caring about this would have unimaginable positive impacts on climate change and our planet. Issues of radicalisation, racism, individualism would be brought to nought. It is the key that can unlock a world of collective action, the positive implications of which are immeasurable. At the very least, we would navigate life in a kinder, gentler way.

Served with Compassion

Niamh Condon

From an early age, I was always looking out for family members, whether that was my brother and sister, my grandmother, who lived nearby, or witnessing my parents visit their older relatives and neighbours. Whether they were helping with odd jobs, or just having a chat and a cup of tea my parents dealt with everyone with compassion and care.

That really stayed with me, and I realised how extremely fortunate I was to have elderly people in my life as I had my grandmother in Ennis and my grandparents in Cork who both played a huge part in my upbringing.

There was my uncle too, who was instrumental in how my career has panned out. He ran a butcher/deli and when I was just twelve, I went to work with him after school and at the weekends. I loved chatting with his older customers. They would tell me how they were going to cook their food and I was only happy to help them with their heavy shopping bags back to their cars or houses. To me, it was all part of the service.

I left school at the age of eighteen and moved from Ennis to study Food Process Engineering in University College, Cork, which was three hours to get to by bus.

This meant that I went to live with my grandparents during those college years. I will forever cherish that time as the three of us developed such a special, bond. Without even thinking about it, I began to cook and care for them while simultaneously they looked after me too.

Those years with my beloved grandparents gave me a

valuable insight into how older people dine, their idiosyncrasies around portions and tastes, and the importance of not wasting food. They consumed food and created meals from the less expensive cuts of meat which when slow cooked gave an incredibly soft texture. This was important for them because they worried that if their food wasn't cooked for hours, it wouldn't be safe. But also, they both wore dentures and couldn't chew on anything too tough.

Respecting their wishes and understanding of their needs helped me to prepare good food and really enjoy mealtimes when we'd sit around the dinner table eating and chatting.

Those conversations inspired me in more ways than I ever thought. Without doubt, they led me to running my own catering company which I found exciting and fast-paced.

But it wasn't until I was asked to work in a nursing home in west Cork that I truly understood the meaning of caring for the elderly. I found a deep passion to provide the best possible care for people who needed my food to survive.

Yet, this wasn't a career move that I'd anticipated and to be honest, I was worried it would stifle my flair for food and that I'd get bored too easily. In fact, the opposite happened.

The brief from the start was simple – cook good fresh food for fifty people in the home, a reasonable request but gradually I realised this was more than just cooking meals for a set number of people every day. This was their home, and I felt a real desire to cook food that would make them feel at home.

All the residents had their own dietary needs and their own stories. I recall one eighty-five-year-old man walking into the kitchen looking for his mother. It was heart-breaking, and I quickly realised, nourishment was more than just plonking meat and two veg on a plate.

I became committed to helping these amazing elderly

people enjoy and savour the food on their plates. Through my research, I discovered that eight per cent of the world's population had a swallowing disorder called 'dysphagia'. This meant that foods needed to be blended and drinks needed to be thickened to enable comfortable safe swallowing.

I realised that when it came to these modified meals, presentation was as important as the food itself. I could not understand how it was ok to blend somebody's meal and then serve it in a coloured bowl to enhance the presentation. Why not enhance the presentation of the food itself, rather than the brown, grey puree which seemed to be the norm. To me, this was unacceptable. I searched for support and training to improve the dining experience for those that I was cooking for. But there was none available, so I set about trying to find ways to do this myself.

I began with small steps, such as separating the ingredients out and blending them individually and then serving the food from ice cream scoops. I would then come out of the kitchen and sit with the residents for meals, so that I could learn what they enjoyed and what worked for them.

It was definitely a learning curve, and I didn't always get it right. I remember one lady who beamed with excitement when she saw the individual scoops of food on her plate. I thought I'd cracked it until she suddenly burst out 'Ice cream!'

This lady had dementia and she recognised the food as ice-cream and therefore expected ice-cream. Because she was on a modified diet with thickened fluids, she was not able to consume ice-cream for safety. My heart sank and I had to go back and rethink how I could change this further.

With simple alterations and listening to the feedback of the care assistants as well as the residents, I was able to improve the presentation. People were now eating more, taking less supplements, and enjoying the food on their plates.

All this allowed me to prepare in advance and have less waste from the kitchen, but I needed support from all involved. I enlisted the help of a dietician to put ourselves in the shoes of those who had a swallowing disorder. We consumed a diet of pureed meals and thickened fluids to understand what the residents were facing. What we learned was that food was more than just nutritional, it was a social activity as well.

I realised how isolating it can feel to try to drink a cup of coffee with a spoon because the consistency had to be thickened. I could understand why some of the residents wanted to dine alone rather than have others see their difficulties with eating.

I was determined to help, so I began to use less of the commercial thickeners available and to instead incorporate the natural thickeners in food to encourage people to eat more.

I was on a mission to share my findings with as many chefs as possible as I knew they too were struggling with modified diets. I have sat with dieticians, doctors, speech and language therapists and asked many questions. As a result, I've built up really good working relationships with the best in the field.

But there is always a need to learn and my passion for wanting to help others led me to go back to my studies, with Food Science being at the forefront. I wanted to be able to understand what happens to the food when you blend it into a puree and digest it. The necessity to ensure that the food that I am preparing is the best nutritional quality for those who consume it is my top priority.

I have recently taken part in a swallow study to understand more about the patient experience for those who may be diagnosed with a dysphagia. I need to have a full understanding of the challenges they face, so that I'm able to prepare excellent quality food and drinks for them.

I've always been a foodie, so it's no surprise that I have

ended up in catering, but I never expected to go down the path I'm on now – a path, it turns out, I'm so passionate about.

And yet, I look back and see the clues were all there, those life affirming meals with my grandparents, the delight I got from working in the deli, and, more recently, the sheer joy of seeing an elderly resident finally tasting and loving the food on their plate after years of struggling to eat.

It has taught me that food served with compassion, empathy and care makes for the perfect recipe. Food is a necessity, not a luxury and everyone should have the right to have a dignified dining experience.

'Our residents do not live in our workplace, we work in their home!'

Empathy in Journalism

Real, Human Stories have the Power to Influence Minds and Motivate Action

Carl O'Brien

One murky afternoon in February, 1966, journalist Michael Viney met with Larry, a thin and frail seventeen-year-old boy.

His mother and father had been 'pretty bad on the drink' and he'd ended up in St Conleth's reformatory school in Co. Offaly two years earlier having been arrested for petty crime.

He spoke of his borrowed clothes and despaired about the 'baldy' haircut he'd just got. There were the multiple floggings, lack of food, fruitless attempts to escape, followed by more beatings, monthly showers. The forced labour in the fields in winter was especially tough with 'so little clothes on you, just the little short coat, and your hands would be just coiled up and you could beat them against a wall and not feel it'.

Of the priests in charge of these institutions, Viney observed: 'These were not the most suitable men to have the care of children', writing that the priests themselves regarded the reformatories as 'places of banishment or refuge for inadequate or misfit religious'.

Viney's series, 'The Young Offenders', published in *The Irish Times* in 1966, exposed the dismal condition of children in institutions.

It would be 2009 before the Ryan report was published, with its scathing findings on abuse of children in orphanages, industrial schools and reformatories. The final report quoted from Viney's series. But in 1966, it was the first time many of the newspaper's affluent readers saw up close the face of the poor, excluded and misunderstood. At a time when many believed such young people were morally inferior and had brought this fate upon themselves, Viney sought to humanise the poor and excluded by eliciting empathy and understanding.

The articles didn't change anything overnight. But, over time, they became a text for sociology students in UCD, led to authorities investigating institutions and contributed to changes which emphasised alternatives to detention and better outcomes for vulnerable young people. It's a reminder that stories – real, human stories – have the power to influence minds and motivate action.

Journalism, at its best, helps to dismantle those social constructions which turn groups of people into 'others' and allows us to view them as different and undeserving. In the right hands, the insight and skill of writers and journalists can make readers identify and empathise with characters in sometimes profound ways.

At its worst, the absence of empathy makes for bad journalism. It facilitates the easy stereotyping of 'welfare cheats', 'illegal immigrants' or 'evil monsters' without exploring their lives; it casts easy and callous judgement on celebrities or politicians without understanding the choices they make. We don't necessarily have to feel sympathy – but it helps to understand people's actions and identify their motivations.

Why are people's stories so powerful? Some academics explain it in terms of 'transportation theory': when you feel so engaged in a story that you feel connected to the character and travel to their world. The more transported you feel, the more likely you'll be to change your opinions about the real world.

I've seen it myself when writing on the lives of asylum seekers living in Ireland's direct provision system. It's a degrading and dehumanising environment where families spend years waiting for their applications to be processed. The system exists on the margins of society, like the industrial schools of old; that distance allows people to cast judgement on those in it without ever understanding the reality of their lives.

I recall interviewing Simmy about what it was to live for years in a caravan, unable to work or cook a meal for her kids because of the direct provision rules; and how her daughter who had sat the Leaving Cert earlier that year would be unable to go to college to study accountancy because she wasn't eligible for free fees. Dozens of other asylum seekers told similar stories of quiet frustration and thwarted ambition in an *Irish Times* series called 'Lives in Limbo'.

A week later, a reader got in contact: he wanted to fund Simmy's daughter to ensure she could go to college; more readers got in contact who wanted to assist others who featured in the series. There were letters to the editor and calls for Dáil debates. Asylum seekers, who realised they had a powerful voice, gathered the courage to speak up and protest. Soon, the Minister for Justice appointed a group to review conditions in the system, which resulted in a report which recommended allowing asylum seekers work, improving supports and speeding up the processing of applications.

Empathy is powerful. Sometimes it can even change a country for the better. Viney was a keen-eyed and empathetic chronicler of Irish life. His social inquiries – into mental illness, single motherhood, care of the elderly, unhappy marriages and more – helped to hold a mirror to a changing Ireland and transported many to places they had never been.

As he later wrote, in a collection of columns to celebrate fifty years in journalism: 'It does seem that in today's Ireland most people now deal with each other more fairly and with greater intelligence and empathy. In today's divided world this can't be bad.'

Green over Blue

Kiernan Forsyth

Being born in to a family of eleven, with eight of them being boys, can be quite formidable. Being the boy that was born the runt of the litter even more so.

Now don't get me wrong, my childhood was tough but amazing, but being consistently reminded of your size did influence my reactions to other people's feelings.

As kids, we had the best of two worlds. On one hand we swam in Sandycove, ran free on Killiney Hill and played football on the streets, and on the other hand went to stay on our uncle's farm to work hard by milking cows, making hay and silage or dipping sheep, and somehow came home feeling we had a holiday. I think moving between these urban and rural settings was an education in itself.

It was when I was twelve in 1972 that I became one of a handful of people in Ireland to receive Growth Hormone Injections. Of course, the standard retort from friends is 'I see they didn't work'. But believe it or not at the time they made me feel Superhero like, a kind of 'Paddy Spiderman'. Feeling like this I began to put myself more in other people's shoes.

Football was my passion and even though I was still quite small I could hold my own at a certain level against the best of them, including my lifelong pal and schoolfriend the legendary footballer Paul McGrath. Going to school and playing football with Paul I did see at times the lack of empathy that was shown to him.

My Dad died when I was fifteen leaving ten children at

home for my Ma to raise. That's when I saw what a real Superhero does. Dad dying when I was so young somehow made me think of pleasing him in things that I would do. Would he or would he not like me to say or do this thing.

Of course, this did not extend to the football field where I developed in to a golfer's worst putt (a nasty little five-footer). I like to think that most of the lads I played with would rather play with me than against me. I then started coaching kids and have done so for over twenty-five years. I quickly realised that to know as much as possible about your players enables you to feel when something is not right. This is every bit as important as developing their skills and creates an atmosphere where different characters can reach their possible potential. Years after coaching players I still get players coming up to me commenting on the great times they had. Of course, you still get the odd, 'I'll never forgive you for dropping me for the Under 16 Final' thrown in for good measure.

At eighteen, I became a postman and from the very start enjoyed it immensely, so much so that forty-two years later I was still doing it. Meeting a big diversity of people on a daily basis I found really enjoyable. Being a small part, and sometimes a big part, of their day.

One time I delivered to a shop that was yards away from the parish church. I would often have a cup of tea with the lady who owned it. One day she asked me to mind the shop for a few minutes. It so happened that mass finished and the shop filled up so I ended up selling the paper or milk to customers whilst at the same time giving them their mail. I realised that this saved me nearly an hour on my delivery time, so as often as I could I would try to make sure I got to the shop before mass ended. Eventually anybody in the area who was waiting on something important in the mail would come down to the shop at mass time.

A time I won't forget was when I was asked by a woman to read to her the contents of a letter. It was from her son in America. I read to her how much he loved her and how much he missed her voice. He wasn't working but was hoping to get something soon and that he was so sorry for the mistakes he had made. He said he hoped and prayed that he would see her again sometime and that she was always in his thoughts. To this day, I still remember the sobs of that woman. We had to hug each other at the end to console ourselves. I still wonder what became of him.

On the Mend

John Gaffey

Take a second to imagine that you're a third-year college student with homicidal tendencies, studying English in the city with your weird roommate, David. He slurps his tea like the cream off a pint and follows it up by clearing the phlegm through his throat – UrghHmmmm. Tolerable, maybe, but after two years with him, you've started to plan his murder. Today was the last straw after a particularly throaty clearing. URGHHMMM. You're going to kill him. Just before you grab the heaviest lamp-shaped object to clatter him with, you remember you've an essay on *Wuthering Heights* due. There's no way you'll manage to read it after the stress of being pre-occupied hiding his body. No, you'll finish the book first. David's demise can wait. While flicking through the pages you get so caught up in the story that you don't even notice the time passing and when you look up again David's taken the 2:23 p.m. train to Cavan for the weekend.

Did reading the book make you a better person? Was the gothic melodrama of Victorian love so heart-wrenching that you went to bed that day with a care for your fellow man that you'll never forget? No.

But that's the impression that people seem to get when I begin to talk about reading with empathy. That if more people could sit down and read a book once in their life, then crime would be replaced with compassion. If this were the case, I would be advocating for our prisons to look more like libraries. Every time I talk to people about my work and what I aim to achieve, the conversation inevitably turns to 'Well which book?' and I can't fault them. Who wouldn't want a book that opens their eyes to all the world's hardships and gave a firm and confident answer on how the reader should act to make everyone's life better? It just doesn't exist. Empathy is, in truth, an uncompromisingly complex emotion and it's not surprising that what has to be done to become more empathetic is equally complex. There just isn't a pill to take before work, or a spray to put on before a date, or a book to read before bed. Being empathetic begins personally and a personal change is glacial.

When I was in secondary school, I don't think I was particularly empathetic. In fact, I'm certain there were things I said and did that were downright unempathetic. Like practising empathy, being young is a painfully slow process. You have nothing figured out. Some hormonal shift occurs where you think growing your hair to your shoulders is a really cool look and you're on the mend from that point on. Likewise, in the same period of my life, I wasn't a reader. This isn't to say I didn't like reading, actually, I did quite a bit. I read the Harry Potter series twice and then fell down the fantasy rabbit hole of reading the Song of Ice and Fire series which, if you didn't know, could save you from a bullet if you put all five thousand pages in your coat pocket. But apart from these two brief obsessions, I didn't do much reading outside of school.

I like to think that changed for me when I was eighteen and stole a copy of *The Great Gatsby* from my school library. Like I said, I was on the mend.

I was at this stage of life where I was becoming very aware of adulthood throttling towards me like a train. It was a feeling that made me look back on the last few years of my life and question where I was going. So, while I was in the library, pretending I had a free class to skip Irish and hiding from a teacher who stalked the hallways looking for stowaways. I had a look at the books around me. I figured the most mature thing you can do in life is read a book. I hadn't quite figured out yet that books could be wonderfully immature when they want to be. I remembered something my dad used to tell me, 'The Great Gaffey is what your granddad called me' and seeing a copy of the book with a Norman Rockwell cover of a man smoking by a yellow jalopy, I seized my chance and pocketed it.

Something about the characters of that book stuck with me, I saw myself in them. When we're talking about empathy, we focus a lot on other people. It's easy to forget that empathy is a lot to do with knowing yourself as well. You understand others when you understand how they're similar to yourself. You feel empathy for others when you understand that a person's reaction to hardship is likely the same as your own. The hurdle comes when we realise that we're similar to everyone, they're all deserving of empathy. Reading gives us a sense of what it's like to be another person, from another world. Their upbringing, class, gender, and outlook can be entirely different from our own. That can be an educating force in its own right, but empathy comes about when we understand that no amount of difference really separates us. I didn't know what it was like to come from the American Midwest or be a bootlegger with a secret identity, but I knew what it was like to want to escape from home and how hard it is to try everything to reach the top and never really be happy.

From that criminal moment, I became a reader.

Since coming to college, I hope I've become more empathetic, finally taking a step that took my whole adolescence to figure out. A step that reading opened for me. I've amassed a modest little shelf of books and lived a modest number of lives through them. I've seen through the eyes of Holocaust survivors, civil rights activists and normal people but I would hesitate to say I understand any of their perspectives. There's a certain power to the word 'understand'. It implies infallibility, that you get it, and it's why for all I believe about the good of reading I'd never dare to say reading is enough. After you put down *To Kill a Mockingbird*, you don't get racialised violence in the American south. You've gotten one perspective on it and you'll need a hundred more and even then, you might not get it. A great deal of harm has been committed by people who thought they understood and it's why we have to remember that books have caused as much hardship in history as they've caused compassion. There's a line to be crossed from empathy in the novel to empathy in the real world and the foundation of that bridge is conversation.

A year and a half ago, I read *The Curious Incident of the Dog in the Night-time*. A story about a young boy with autism struggling to cope with his parent's divorce. I had a friend with autism in one of my classes at the time and something possessed me to ask him if he knew of the book, and if so, what he thought of it. He didn't, but it sparked a conversation about what it's like to be neural atypical in a world that moves faster than some can cope with. A lot of the time these stories that focus on the experiences of people outside of the cultural norm only make waves once they become movies. The usual idea about how the book was better than the film applies to empathy. The empathy was better. At the same time though, the empathy you're going to practise from sitting down and talking to someone will be miles more advanced than just reading about people. Reading just happens to be one of those things that gives us a bit of confidence to talk about something that we wouldn't know how to address otherwise.

As I said, there's no one book. Not every story is going to

have what's necessary to make someone empathetic. Not every person is going to have an empathetic response to the same story. What matters more than only reading the right books is that you pick up books as quickly as you put them down and read them thoughtfully. That you think about what you've read and how it applies to your own life. How were you able to tell what a side character was feeling in a book without it being laid out for you? That's empathy. Why did Arthur Weasley going to hospital break your heart as if he was your own goofy Dad? That's empathy. Why did you spend a day reading about Emmett Till after reading THUG? That's empathy. Each book pushes you just another inch forward to a cliff-edge where you figure it out. That this story is fiction, but its world is a fact, and only you can change it.

The Person who Sees

Ailbhe Greaney

As a photographer and academic, I have come to understand the power that looking allows. It is an essential element of empathetic exchange. Within this looking, it is often photography that allows us to see. To see both oneself and another person. Becoming a photographer is a long slow process, a durational commitment. We often think of a photograph as fleeting, a single moment captured by a sensitive surface. But where does this sensitivity lie? Within the silver halide crystals found in the physicality of film or the sensitised silicon wafer of digital technology? It lies within both of these surfaces. Most significantly and ultimately, however, it lies within ourselves. The person who sees.

Before light can act photographically, it must first act upon us, the human beings whose actions connect light with the sensitive surface of photographic technology. We are the original sensitive surface, the mechanism through which all images are filtered. From the moment we are born, we embark upon a lifetime of sensitisation and de-sensitisation. Our ability to see ourselves and to see others is shaped by experiences – views that continually expand or block our understanding of the world. Not even 200 years old, yet older still as a concept, photography's technology and identity are now inextricably linked to our own. Its form, its function is woven into the fabric of our landscape. It has become an extension of our own body, ourselves, our identity. A complex medium, even the very date of its invention is contested.

The very first image to be permanently rendered within the camera obscura, to be fixed, was entitled 'View from the Window at Le Gras', taken in 1826 by Niecephore Niepce. The term 'fixed' is used here because the mechanism for capturing an image existed long before the fixing of Niepce's view. The first reference to the camera obscura was by Giovanni Battista della Porta in his book *Natural Magic* in 1558. As such, it was possible to conceive of the view that the contemporary camera would provide long before the fixed photograph actually existed. The camera obscura was first used during a time when such an apparatus would have been considered a thing of magic. Those inside the camera obscura, or dark chamber, were concealed from view and the perspective that this camera afforded – projected onto the inside of the box as an inverted image via a small aperture or hole in the wall – was a secretive glimpse onto the world outside the box. As such, the dream of photography existed long before the technology could 'fix' an image or a view and make it permanent. Even Niepce's view, rendered onto a pewter place, was not a permanent solution and could not be sufficiently replicated. Further attempts to render an image were too weak to produce the necessary etching from the original pewter plate. The exposure time for 'View from Le Gras' was approximately eight hours, during this time the sun moved from east to west and as such, appears to shine on both sides of the building. Thereby revealing an impossible view.

An unskilled draftsman, Niepce sought to use the camera obscura to record what he saw, believing that it might be possible to make the trace of light projected into the camera obscura permanent. Unfortunately, for Niepce, his invention was not secure enough to be accepted by society at large and he died before photography was formally recognised via Fox Talbot's photogenic drawings in 1834 and the Daguerreotype in 1839. In 1839, Fox Talbot, working with Sir John Herschel, discovered a way to make more secure or permanent the photographic image using hyposulphate, a method that is still used today as a fixer for black and white images in the darkroom. Talbot, hearing word of Daguerre's invention in France rushed to release news of his own process to the world via the Royal Society in Britain, ahead of Daguerre. Niepce's process was the precursor for all of this, and his view is recognised as the first photograph, collected by Helmut Gernsheim and donated to the Harry Ransom Center in Austin, Texas, in 1963, having gone missing in 1905. Niepce's 'point de vue' is an example of his Héliographie process or 'sun writing' , and, as described by the Harry Ransom Center, it reveals 'an image of the rooftops and trees visible from his studio window'.*

The dream of representing one's own view was made real and permanent via these discoveries. The long cultivation of this dream accounts for the rapid acceleration of photographic technology since these dates of invention. Once 'fixed', however, photographic technology has set about repeatedly 'unfixing' itself by its continual evolution as both a medium, technology and concept. Ironically photographic and video communication used within networks such as Instagram, Snapchat and TikTok, are generated to both appear and disappear, they are transient, much like early photographic images whose sensitive surface could not be fixed prior to 1839. As such, photography acts a way of thinking, a way of responding to society and the demands and peculiarities of its time.

Pressing the button of a camera or camera phone is an action that can be and has been automated, mechanised, weaponised. From its inception, photography has been utilised

---

* 'The Niépce Heliograp', Harry Rasom Center, The University of Texas at Austin, accessed 30 March 2022, https://www.hrc.utexas.edu/niepce-heliograph/.

as a means of identification – of difference, of sameness – of sameness in difference – of difference in sameness. The view from the camera can be dehumanised and desensitised by over exposure, by the attempt to 'other' and to differentiate so as to disconnect. The view from the camera also has the power, the incredible power, to connect.

With empathy, this power can be harnessed. Photography's very subjective nature masquerading within a seemingly objective technology makes it a vital tool in the representation of ALL human form. Its own ubiquitous form means that it is a technology that lives with us. Unlike many other forms of expression, it crosses all aspects of our lives, from the gallery wall to the book, the magazine, the billboard – to the computer screen and the phone. Young people now use photography within the context of social media networks as a tool for communication, as essential as the spoken or written word. Certain research suggests, however, that an overload of contact through social networks – especially in the context of COVID 19 – as well as a high level of intolerance for uncertainty, has led to an increase in anxiety within young people.[†] In relation to the written word, we know when we cannot read its form, conversely, we do not necessarily know that we cannot read the form of a photograph. This kind of potential visual illiteracy within a culture outpaced by its transformative imaging technologies, needs to be addressed with regard to the contemporary use of photography as language; with the power to both connect and disconnect, to make certain and uncertain, to fix and to unfix.

The island of Ireland is politically, if not geographically, young. Just 100 years in its current state, its contemporary fragile peace has now been jeopardised by the complexities of Brexit

† F Glowacz, E Schmits, 'Psychological distress during the COVID-19 lockdown: The young adults most at risk', *Psychiatry Research,* vol. 293 (Nov 2020): 113486. doi: 10.1016/j.psychres.2020.113486.

and it is faced with a subsequent crisis of national identity. In addition, the context of COVID 19, within which the essential physical socialisation of our young has been compromised, requires that we strive even harder to understand the way in which young people and such young identities communicate, socialise and empathise through the image as disseminated by new technological and social media platforms. Photographic technology is young too, relative to other forms of expression. Such a tool, such magic, in both the realm of close-up magic and photographic magic, 'is a multisensory experience that calls – instantaneously and without our consciously knowing it – upon our capacity to script our own sense of visual reality'.[‡]

Within this context, we must ask how are young people scripting their own sense of reality, using the tools of photography and social media in the context of the twenty-first century?

As a young person, my own sense of reality and identity has been inextricably linked to photography and, to reference the art critic John Berger, to ways of seeing.[§] In 2000, I was presented with a Fulbright Award by Nobel Prize Winner John Hume, Senator George Mitchell and Loretta Brennan Glucksman in Dublin Castle. Along with a number of other generous bursaries, awards and the incalculable kindness and generosity of my parents and family, this allowed me to begin a three-year MFA Degree in Photography and Related Media at the School of Visual Arts New York. For myself then, moving to New York in 2000 as a student of photography, with 9/11 striking the city a year later, my own photographic work had at its origin a desire to both see and replicate or duplicate the world as I once knew it or wished it to be. In this way photographs have, to reference curator and critic John

‡ Charlotte Cotton, *Photography Is Magic* (New York: Aperture, 2015), 1.
§ John Berger, *Ways of Seeing* (London: Penguin, 1972).

Szarkowski, served as windows , offering a view onto both the known and the unknown, often taken with eyes closed as much as open.¶ Originally from Galway, I was twenty-one at the time of leaving, and if my work has been an attempt to fill a gap, it has also operated to create a gap within the image plane.

I experienced an absence of place borne out of the absence of family, within a city as great and tumultuous as New York. It was photography, the act of looking, seeing – slowly over time – that allowed me to first understand aspects of what is invisible and often unknowable. To understand those displaced not just externally, but also internally. On 11 September 2001, I remember the twin towers covered. A bright sky turned grey. The early morning streets at once empty and then suddenly thick with the helpless. Most of all I remember that in New York, and sometimes in crisis, help comes as wordless action. On that day, I was cloaked within an instantaneous shroud of physical friendship. New friends from far flung places we watched the city from its hills, absorbing the crash. I remember the sound of new voices talking to one another, faces turned towards each other silently. Time seemed extended and, in the slowness, we saw each other as individuals within the mass.

My own photographic practice has come to centre around themes of migration and the definition of home in an expanded field, encompassing notions of the marginal and the intellectual exile. Again, this practice has developed slowly over time. As has the act of looking and seeing. A former teacher and mentor, Stephen Shore, speaks of seeing with conscious attention. Shore believes that photography is a tool for learning how to do that, something which can be of benefit to anyone. He has said that 'seeing with conscious attention, and seeing with self-awareness, in a way feeds people, feeds part of the mind'.**

¶ John Szarkowski, *Mirrors and Windows* (New York: MOMA, 1978).

** '*Stephen Shore | HOW TO SEE*', Museum of Modern Art, accessed 30 March

As a student, I spent months printing the archive of trauma that resulted in the photographic exhibition 'Here is New York: a democracy of photographs'; as an empathetic response to 9/11. Image after image unfolded as individuals – from survivors, fire fighters to established photographers – began to understand this crisis, this trauma, by looking, by seeing themselves in each other and by using the camera as a means by which to navigate the unknown. In 2015, then an academic, I was with students during the November Paris attacks. Here, I was able to provide some of the support that was both present and absent for myself during 9/11; a time when technology was not able to act as a support mechanism and communication was less reliable. As a founding member and Director of the BA (Hons) Photography & Video Degree (2007) and MFA Photography Degree (Campus 2010/ E-Learning 2015) at Ulster University's Belfast School of Art, I have been working slowly with young students since 2007 in a post conflict Belfast. The ability of these young people to use photography to understand themselves and each other is continually inspiring. Their lives are young, but the legacy they have been left is long and runs deep. Social media and photography as a form of expression and representation have allowed such young people to cross hard lines of sectarian divide. Photography has historically acted as a portal, allowing us entry to worlds beyond our own. Used as a form of communication and within art practice, it now allows us to cross walls at the end of our garden. In the context of Belfast, these walls are sometimes Peace Walls or Peace Lines. The virtual has the potential to enter the real, allowing young people to see and to know those who they have been separated from by lines drawn by others.

The fast-paced connections created through systems of social

2022, https://www.moma.org/calendar/exhibitions/3769.

media have the ability to both alienate and authenticate one's sense of self. Photography's unfixed nature and fluidity speaks to, and parallels, young people's desire to resist definition – to be non-binary, non-sectarian, multi-cultural. Without some sense of self however, such lives are at risk of manipulation, of being used in the service of those with a more powerful agenda, where seeing is not to look and to look is very often not to see. To see with conscious attention is to engage empathetically with others. To look for the beauty in difference, and the gesture of sameness. We are all linked by our peculiarity, very often our only point of connection is our difference. Photography allows us to look directly at that difference, and to know it as our own.

Empathy, Images and the Internet

Mary McGill

The great art critic John Berger once wrote, 'Every image embodies a way of seeing'. As a media studies lecturer and writer, I think about Berger's words a great deal. Most especially, I think about what they have to teach us in an age of rapidly evolving digital technologies that have enabled the proliferation of visual media as never before.

We live now in a world of images, those made by others and those of our own making. Like all forms of media, images can be powerful vessels for truth. They can help us understand issues far removed from our own lives, creating the conditions for empathy. But images can also have the opposite effect.

Images can be used to humiliate, violate and 'other'. Images can obscure and mislead; they can outright lie. As advocates of media literacy point out, such is the power of images, and humanity's desire for them, we need to learn how to treat them critically.

I am of the last generation that can remember analogue life, when photographs were mainly taken at special occasions; given the costs involved they were printed sparingly and collected in albums and frames designed to last a lifetime, perhaps longer.

Now photographic images are everywhere, so plentiful as to be disposable, forgettable, an everyday activity rather than a special one. We no longer need to print them; our phones and 'clouds' do the storing. Images have become less precious in the sense that they are so easily and cheaply created and more precious in the way they purport to represent us in the digital world of the internet, a space that in a very short time has transformed how we live our lives.

On social media, we use images to express ourselves, to have conversations, to cultivate an idea of who we are that appeals to others and to ourselves. But this proliferation of images can obscure as much as it can shed light. One only has to glance at a platform like Instagram to observe that our new ability to create images can breed conformity rather than creativity.

On digital platforms, conventions set down by culture and what technology prioritises act as a lens through which we are invited to see ourselves and others. This way of seeing, usually guided by norms long associated with fashion and beauty photography and stereotypes of race, class and gender, can produce effects that are alienating.

Platforms that encourage judgemental gazing – and most of them do, it is what ranking mechanisms such as 'likes' and 'comments' are all about – invite the user to scrutinise not only others but themselves. In these environments, images are commodities; they can be used to gain status through visibility, social approval and the amassing of followers. In learning to 'see' ourselves as images, we risk being absorbed into a system of commodification where we rank ourselves and each other as if we are objects, not people.

Berger's point speaks as much about what images do not show as what they do. However beautiful or shocking or profound, an image or a photograph is only ever partial. It can never fully capture a human being in all their strength, vulnerability and complexity nor can it fully capture context. All of us are more than the images that are taken to stand for us. But viewing the world and each other through a screen every day can do strange things to our minds. We can make the mistake of reducing others to the level of image. We can use people's images against them. We can forget that behind every image, no matter how perfect, 'ugly' or annoying, is a person as real and as complicated as we are.

In her reflections on the nature of evil, the philosopher Hannah Arendt argued that empathy requires the ability to think for oneself so as not to fall into the trap of letting others do our thinking for us. As she saw it, if we cannot think critically about the world and our place in it, we cannot imagine, and without imagination, empathy is impossible.

In the digital age, we have a duty to think critically about 'the ways of seeing' encouraged by social media, which rely so heavily on judgement and external validation. A human being is more than an image; we should never be mistaken one for the other. On platforms that can make empathy difficult, reminding ourselves that we are all so much more than pixels on screen can be a simple but powerful way to practise it.

Empathy for the Devil ... and the Nuns

Mark Brennan

For as long as I can remember, I never got on well with nuns. Some saw them as holy and pious. I saw devils. That's right. I said it. Right or wrong, I despised nearly all of them. They felt the same about me. I'm not sure when we reached this agreement, but it was very, very early on. Almost certainly from the earliest of primary school. From there we were set. Somehow, I always felt they were a sham. Like bad cops, abusive priests, and others we've come to realise exist in our midst. They were the majority of my teachers, and a good part of my social world for all of my childhood and early youth.

I saw the nuns in three types: the holy, the lost and the vicious:

The Holy: An extremely small number were miraculous. Not because of their faith, but because of their actions. They were simply exceptional human beings acting to make the world better. For all, religion was a minor characteristic – at best, the small backdrop for positive lives well lived. Advancing humanity with empathy was their trade.

The Lost: The majority of the nuns were indifferent, distant and detached. Many were brilliant – significantly gifted in music, art and other areas. Really truly exceptional! I remember Sister Michelangelo an amazingly accomplished musician. In another world, she would have been on Broadway, filling arenas, touring the world. Many of the 'lost' were prone to anger, and what I would now recognise as depression. It was the kind of anger and depression that comes from knowing the Eden that you've been denied. And while large in numbers, the 'lost' never intervened in the actions of the vicious.

The Vicious: A small group were monsters and vicious, hiding behind the impervious protection of the habit. They were abusive, torturous and violent on all levels. Much like we've seen with church scandals in recent decades, true monsters are expertly skilled in placing themselves in religious orders for the cover they provide. The Vicious existed in large numbers, and their impacts were massive on the generations left under their care.

These nuns were part of the Order of the Blessed Virgin Mary (the BVMs!). For reference, I would put them up against the Christian Brothers any day. I often wonder what a title match between the two would look like. Both taught maths … and how to take a punch.

But enough of the sob stories. This essay is not about wrongs done or perceived. It's about how empathy brings disparate people together and allows us to deeply understand each other.

In a true twist of fate, despite being turned off education at an early age, I became a teacher and a researcher. Even more bizarre, I ended up in academia. One of my first gigs was at a university 'affiliated' with the BVMs. Upon arrival, I learned that the university was more than affiliated. This was the corporate headquarters, the mothership, the place where nuns began, where some were allowed to stay and teach/research … and where they came to live out their final years on campus or in an adjacent BVM retirement home. I was outnumbered 1,000 to 1, and the battle between us was back on! I had scores to settle!

But almost immediately, empathy intervened. Twenty plus years on, I encountered many of the nuns that I had in primary/secondary school. The ones that were holy were still godly, enlightened, complete and peaceful people. They had chosen wisely – the calling – teacher, faith, or whatever it might be. Bless them.

I found that the vicious were still vicious but had faded in their intensity. Perhaps, in their older age, they had come to terms with some of their previous sins or ghosts. Perhaps a diet of rage can't be sustained over a lifetime.

With the nuns that I had thought of as the Lost, empathy shone most bright. They were far more complex than my simple description. Again, Michelangelo reappeared. I would run into her at various campus events and quickly casual chats turned into profound discussions. We would share coffees, teas and the occasional whiskey. Increasingly she provided her take on all those years ago. She pulled in others who shared their stories.

Most recounted being young women in their twenties and early thirties. Many were either forced into the nunnery or had mistakenly chosen this path thinking it would fulfil their faith and identity. Several remarked that by the time they realised this was not their best path, it was too late. Getting out, while technically possible, was not a real option. Leaving meant being ostracised by family and faith. Leaving meant entering another world they were unprepared for and largely did not know. They were stuck, trapped and there was no getting out. They adjusted as best they could.

All told stories of routinely being transferred to other parishes every three to four years. Being disconnected from families, in an environment where long-term friendships were hard to forge, and often being assigned to what they viewed as remote rural outposts (like my homeplace) was devastating. It was a foreign, stifling and lonely world for them. From an empathetic perspective, this had to be incredibly hard for young people faced with a life they didn't expect or really want. Considering how difficult I can become, having been away from my wife and friends/family after a month or two away, I recognise how hard life was for these nuns. I'm certain I would have behaved far worse than they did.

Some were LGBTQ+ who in their youth saw few opportunities to be who they are or live the life they wanted. The convent was one of very few options for a life devoid of questions about career, marriage and children. It would be assumed that joining the order was purely a religious calling, not a shelter in a society that would shun them. While the convent was not a place to find a partner for most, miracles did occur for others. It was a safe setting where they met the true love of their lives. Nonetheless, religious life often resulted in the frequent transfers to other parishes for years on end. They would be geographically separated from life partners, not knowing when, or if, they might be together again.

For this latter group, I think about my relationship with my wife and how central it was to my own personal and psychological development in my twenties and thirties. I became an infinitely better person because of her and the lives we experienced together. I can't imagine the character I would be if we had been forced to live separate lives – for years on end – during such an important part of our lives. These nuns had to endure that awfulness.

The ability of empathy to open up understanding in this setting was unique. Again, this was the mothership of the BVMs. There were few secrets there, and while not commented on, it was common for couples to live openly together. They shared apartments, some had their own homes adjacent to campus, they had their meals together, they walked together each night around the neighbourhood, had friends over for meals and wished each other off in the mornings for work. After many years of separation, challenges and all else, they were complete.

It's funny how when we take on empathy that our entire understanding of the world can change dramatically. Today I see the nuns simply as people trying to make the most of what they could with a life they found themselves in. Not saints or devils, but common human beings. I'm still not sure what they think of me!

Educating for and with Empathy

The Role of Empathy in Teacher Education

Niamh Flynn and Emer Davitt

Empathy has been an increasingly distinct element of our efforts to cope with the unique and unprecedented challenges of the COVID-19 crisis. Throughout these turbulent times, we have become very familiar with the mantra of 'being kind to each other', and have encountered or directly participated in other-oriented and prosocial acts such as whole communities mobilising to provide supports to vulnerable groups. Additionally, it was suggested that empathy for vulnerable members of society was one of the key factors underlying the motivation to adhere to physical distancing; the public health counter-measure which became the centre-point of our lived experience of the pandemic. Direct observation of the importance of empathy for everyday survival and unity during this period of uncertainty has shone a spotlight on potential pathways to increased levels of empathy among society in general, and in particular, among adolescents, who are developmentally primed for the growth of empathy. Here we consider the role of teacher education in growing the capacity and commitment of educators to foster an empathy-centred curriculum and culture in second-level schools; an approach that we believe will contribute to the creation of a more inclusive, compassionate and just future society.

Despite most of us feeling that we have a general sense of what empathy is, there is very considerable debate among academic researchers across different disciplines as to the true nature of the phenomenon. However, some commonality is evident across definitions in the form of two central dimensions; cognitive empathy (perceiving and understanding the perspective and feelings of another), and affective empathy (joining with them in these feelings whilst being aware of the source of the feelings). This broad framing differentiates empathy from sympathy, with the distinction between the two being akin to feeling *as* versus feeling *for* the person. Interestingly, it is believed that empathy does not always require a direct physical encounter with a person; rather, it can also be evoked for a real, yet distant, person who is verbally described, and even for fictional or imaginary characters.

An increasing body of neuroscience research suggests that there is a neurological basis for empathy. This is linked to mirror neurons in a part of the brain called the anterior cingulate cortex that have been found to become activated in response to both personally experienced pain and observed pain in others. However, whilst discussions about neural pathways appear to suggest an automatic, involuntary basis to empathy, it is believed that empathy is in fact malleable. That is, we can bring empathy under conscious control through a variety of cognitive process like focusing attention on the other person, and physical processes such as distancing ourselves from the other person; all of which either increase or decrease our likelihood of experiencing and expressing empathy. Furthermore, a considerable amount of research in psychology has highlighted that empathy can fluctuate very significantly depending on dynamic interpersonal factors including how similar the person is to ourselves, what our current mood is, how much we value the person, how many needs and how much power we perceive the person to have, and what our cognitive load is (i.e., how much is on our mental workbench at that particular point in time). Accordingly, an emerging view in psychology is that it is more accurate to think of empathy not as an inherent and fixed ability that a person either possesses or lacks, but alternatively as an interpersonal process that results from the interplay of stable and temporary factors across the empathiser and empathisee. However, a reasonable question is: if empathy is so hard to get a handle on, why does it continue to enthral so many people across different walks of life? The likely answer is that empathy has been found to be predictive of, or at the very least associated with, an impressive array of extremely desirable individual and group life outcomes. These include increased social competence, reduced prejudice, increased sensitivity and commitment to social justice, reduced conflict across different social groups, reduced anti-social behaviour, reduced aggression, increased pro-social behaviour, and improved physical and psychological health.

Adolescence is believed to be a critical time for the development of empathy, which is viewed as a pivotal social skill with implications for how individuals respond to local and global social justice issues both at a young age, and into and throughout adulthood. Indeed, empathy in young people has been found to be linked to reduced levels of bullying, improved social and cognitive adjustment, and increases in responsible civic behaviour into the future. Due to these developmental trends, combined with research evidence suggesting that empathy is a malleable capacity that can be turned on and enhanced, it is not surprising that empathy has become an important focus in schools. Educators have started to explore educating for empathy through implementation of training interventions such as the Activating Social Empathy programme that has been developed by researchers at the UNESCO Child and Family Research Centre at the University of Galway and the UNESCO Chair in Community, Leadership, and Youth Development at the Pennsylvania State University in conjunction with Foróige.

Programmes of this nature aim to empower and support young people in developing and enhancing their empathy skills, thereby increasing their readiness and motivation to become more pro-socially and civically engaged within their communities. Since empathy education holds considerable promise for improving multiple learning and general life outcomes for young people and by extension, those in their communities, it is our strong belief that teacher education courses should prioritise exposure of future teachers to the philosophy, research bases and methods of school-based empathy training programmes.

A less direct, but nonetheless powerful, school-based pathway to enhanced levels of empathy in society is educating with empathy. It is our view, and the view of many teacher educators, that empathy enables teachers to better recognise and understand the needs and strengths of students, families and communities, especially if they are teaching in racially, culturally and linguistically diverse settings. In addition, an empathic disposition on the part of a teacher is often associated with a strengthened commitment to exploring and addressing social justice issues with their students. Additionally, empathy is seen as a crucial element of positive teacher-student relationships. The famous psychologist, Carl Rogers, writing in 1969, urged that teaching should be grounded in supportive, non-directive and empathic relationships with students. He proposed that relationships of this nature could be achieved through realness or genuineness in interactions with students, unconditional positive regard (which he described as accepting the learner for who they are, and trusting their ability to develop and learn), and through efforts to see the world through the learner's eyes after deep and active listening.

Despite that fact that teacher-student interactions are less intense, less direct and more transitory than those with adult caregivers, relationships with teachers are nonetheless highly significant in helping young people to develop emotional security, which sets the scene for greater engagement with learning. Further, positive teacher-student relationships are believed to be particularly influential for students who have multiple risk factors in their lives, to the extent that they may even compensate for family and educational disadvantage. Some of the outcomes that have been found in research to be associated with high quality teacher-student relationships at primary and secondary level include increased levels of academic engagement and performance, attendance and social-emotional adjustment, and reduced levels of disruptive behaviour, suspension and school drop-out. Positive teacher-student relationships also yield benefits for teachers themselves, ranging from increases in job satisfaction, positive emotions and feelings of efficacy, to lower levels of emotional exhaustion and stress. Indeed, positive relationships with students are frequently cited by teachers as one of the primary reasons for entering the profession, and subsequently, one of the principal sources of enjoyment and motivation during teaching.

Based on these persuasive research-based findings, encouraging future teachers to develop an empathic disposition is increasingly becoming an explicit goal of teacher education despite an otherwise packed curriculum for training. Many teacher educators, including ourselves, perceive empathy as an essential resource that should be cultivated and strengthened during the initial teacher education years for the ultimate wellbeing of children, young people and wider society. To this end, during professional training, the deeply embedded care ethic that many individuals who choose teaching as a career already possess is shaped and deepened. Trainee teachers are encouraged and supported to espouse and display concern, open-mindedness, curiosity, warmth, empathy, honesty, trust and respect in all interactions with their students. They are empowered to apply inclusive teaching practices that reach and support all students, particularly those at the edges of the classroom. They are challenged to be available to their students – to have sustained, authentic yet appropriately boundaried interactions that do not terminate rigidly at the sound of the class bell. In essence, they develop the confidence to be real and approachable for their students, and to regard personalising or humanising encounters as a bridge to relatedness rather than mistakes that undermine their authoritative presence in the classroom. Most importantly, they are inspired to strive towards the development of safe shared spaces in their classrooms, where they can listen deeply, ask questions and learn from their students. In this way, future teachers are empowered to begin the important process of acquiring students' cultural and social perspectives; to begin to see the world through the unique lens of their students.

We end this piece with the inspiring practice-based reflections of a number of our trainee teachers about the importance of empathy in education.[††]

> It is essential to listen in order for empathy to be promoted in the class. It is important to reject stereotypes in the classroom and value each student's difference, and to encourage the students to deviate from in-group bias, and establish a compass to empathise with people outside of their social circles and the wider world.

> In my school placement this year, I see how a good relationship can be built around empathy. In teaching with empathy, I actively listen to my students and reflect on what I hear. I make more of a conscious effort to cater to their needs, rather than just getting

†† Sincere thanks to newly qualified teachers, Zoe Bourke (excerpt 1) and Shauna Lyons (excerpt 2), for granting permission to quote their insightful reflections on empathy created during their training in the School of Education at the University of Galway.

> through lessons. By intentionally focusing on students' needs, my students and I have created a more positive and safer learning environment in which everyone is given the chance to grow and develop. Naturally, I don't have much input in unit or curricula planning. However, by modelling empathy in my own behaviour, I hope this inspires students to do the same.

Hearing these committed, empathic and caring voices, we are very optimistic for both the educators of the future and the young people whose lives they will impact. An empathic school culture extending outwards is undoubtedly something for us all to strive for in our work with young people.

YHTAPME

Dedicated to Mike

Róisín Hanley

A Little Girl was sat in her big sister's bedroom next to her Mum and Dad.

There they were, hand-in-hand, and about to tell her the biggest news she had ever received.

'You have a different way of seeing, thinking and understanding to others,' they said. 'You have Dyslexia'.

'I have Dyslexium?'

'No Love, Dyslexia.'

The Little Girl cried in confusion and fear and wondered why she had to be different to others. She knew she wasn't alone, however, as Dad also had dyslexium – oh wait no, dyslexia.

But the thought of the dreaded weekly spelling tests at school were always too much, even if Dad himself had always managed, and did well (in spite of the spelling errors). Other little girls looked forward to Fridays, but not this Little Girl. Fridays meant fear; fear of failure.

Though the Little Girl survived Fridays and each of the day's spelling tests, her worries were not over. When she finally came home, a little red book, *Toe by Toe* (A Highly Structured Multi-Sensory Reading Manual for Teachers and Parents), would serve to remind her that she had – as Mum and Dad had said – a different way of seeing, thinking and understanding to others.

The Little Girl sat at the big kitchen table with *Toe by Toe,* sussing and sounding big words – ones she had never seen or even tried to say before. Mum sat across with an encouraging smile and a hand squeeze. She was full of empathy for every word that the Little Girl fumbled and faltered on. Every squeeze told the Little Girl that her Mum believed in her and was here, and this was the only thing the Little Girl needed.

Back in school, a well-intentioned teacher asked the Little Girl to read aloud as Gaeilge, as she did with every other child. Teacher knew better than anyone that the Little Girl was, in fact, very bright. However, in her eagerness to encourage the Little Girl to confront her fears, Teacher didn't wholly consider the Little Girl's different way of seeing, thinking and understanding. *Toe by Toe* didn't teach the Little Girl how to read as Gaeilge, but reading aloud *as Gaeilge* taught the Little Girl a hard lesson: not everyone would be there for an empathetic hand squeeze when she read, like Mum always was. As she began to speak, the Little Girl stumbled and fumbled like never before. When she paused, she heard a sound that would ring in her ears long after it had finished. She looked up from her book to witness a display of judgement from her classmates who, as of yet, had not been taught much about empathy. A Little Boy was sniggering at the Little Girl while she struggled. This Little Boy then found himself triggering a painful feeling he did not intend to cause.

The Little Girl blushed from her head to her toes and wept bitterly, and longed to be somewhere else. Teacher scolded the boy and offered a kind-hearted hug for the Little Girl, who now bore a cut caused by insensitivity; a cut that wasn't going away anytime soon. The scolding did not make the Little Girl feel any better, however, as she knew deep down that the Little Boy did not understand how her dyslexia affected her and, if he had, he would not have ridiculed her. Instead, he would have empathised with her.

This was the first of many belittling experiences that the

Little Girl would undergo as a result of her dyslexia. This spectre of rejection would follow her, even though all she did differently was see, think and understand.

The Little Girl continued her journey through school with dyslexia, and many days ended in tears of confusion and fear. While her different perspective seemed enormous at times, when the Little Girl didn't think too deeply about it, the biggest obstacle her dyslexia presented alone was the confusion of b's and d's.

Those pesky b's and d's, the Little Girl would think, how unfair that they look the exact same to in my eyes and no one else's.

Her worst nightmare used to be those dreaded Friday tests, but that was no longer the Little Girl's biggest concern. She was experiencing something much more nerve-wrecking going on in her life – something that was called bullying, as she would later discover. This came from one particular bully who used the Little Girl's dyslexia against her. Every Friday, before 9 o'clock, the bully would ask the girl to spell aloud every word that was due to appear on the test. The Little Girl would stammer and struggle while the bully seized her chance to be cruel, both verbally and physically. The wounds the Little Girl already bore from previous insensitivity to her difficulties were worsened by this bully, who could not have truly understood how her actions affected others.

It was not all bad, however. The Little Girl had a Neighbour her age who would sometimes help her before the Friday test. Running to her Neighbour's house, filled with the excitement of seeing a friend, was always something that consoled her.

The Little Girl and her Neighbour would begin to practise the words in the books. The first time they practised, fear stormed the Little Girl's heart, as previous episodes of fumbling and stumbling resulted in suffering. As she began to read aloud in front of her Neighbour, the inevitable happened: the Little Girl confused the spellings of there, their and they're. She prepared for a hit, shut her eyes and held her breath … but nothing happened. The Little Girl slowly opened one eye to see her Neighbour smiling and with her hand out saying 'they always confuse me too, we can learn them together'.

The Little Girl was shocked that the Neighbour responded with such empathy and kindness to her as, before this, the only person who had showed her true compassion was her family. This made the Little Girl wonder why some classmates and friends showed empathy, when others, like her bully, enjoyed making those around them feel powerless. This didn't make much sense to the Little Girl when she was small, but it would soon become clearer when she became a teenager.

The Little Girl was now a Teenager, and started Secondary School. Her Secondary School was sat atop a big hill that seemed far away. It wasn't really far, but it was far from what she knew, as not many of her friends were joining her there. This turning point marked the beginning of a new set of challenges for the Teenager.

The Teenager never coped well with change, and this was the biggest change she had experienced yet. Although one thing did remain the same in a way; there was a Resource room and a Resource Teacher, similar to primary school where the once Little Girl would go with another child who shared her perspective to a space specifically for them. A Safe Space, the Little Girl then, and the Teenager now, thought. But the Teenager soon realised that the Resource Teacher would make an impact in her life far beyond teaching.

Resource periods happened during different times each day,

and each time was the Teenager's favourite part of the day. The Teenager would wait with excitement until the clock struck the hour and she would dart down the hallway, towards her safe space and towards happiness.

Her differences would seem enormous again when, one day, the Teenager was leaving her regular classroom for Resource Time and a fellow student asked, 'where are you going?' The Teenager responded innocently, 'to the Resource Room!' The other student smirked and replied with a familiar callousness that the Teenager had not experienced in some time: 'oh, the room where the stupid people go'.

This felt like a lower blow than the Teenager had ever experienced, as another person had said the exact words she told herself any time she mispronounced or misspelt a word. The Teenager in that moment accepted that she was a stupid person.

The Resource Teacher could see the teenager wasn't her usual self after this incident, and asked her what the matter was. The Teenager couldn't lie and brush it off, she didn't have her family or her Neighbour with her, and the only person she could turn to was the Resource Teacher. The Teenager trusted her, so she decided to tell the Resource Teacher everything she had gone through and was feeling about herself and others. After the first few words came out of her mouth, tears began to spill everywhere.

The Resource Teacher, equipped with experience and empathy, comforted the Teenager and said, 'the student doesn't understand what dyslexia is, what you work through everyday, because if they did know, they would be treating you with respect and empathy. They would understand that all you do differently is see, think and understand. Dyslexia would never make anyone more or less stupid, if anything it makes you braver and smarter because it forces you to overcome.

Compassion and caring doesn't come naturally to some people, but over time it can be taught and understood.'

The Resource Teacher continued to help the Teenager through six whole years without judgement and always taught the Teenager not to dwell on what people falsely presumed about her dyslexia. In doing so, she taught the teenager to believe in herself and to lead by example in showing kindness and empathy towards others.

Through its total absence in some experiences that cut her to the core, and through its immense presence in other situations that encouraged and moved her utterly, the importance of Empathy was made known to the Teenager. By the time she became a woman, she understood that Empathy is what makes us human.

The Little Girl, the Teenager and now, the woman, is the author of this chapter. My name is Róisín Hanley. My experiences of other people showing and withholding empathy have moulded me into the person I am today. My dyslexia has never stopped me from achieving everything I've wanted and the people around me have created a beautiful safe space for empathy to be in the surrounding. I am a recent graduate of a Bachelor of Arts degree in Children Studies at the University of Galway, as well as my final year in a Certificate of Ballet Teaching Studies with the Royal Academy of Dance, London.

I hope this Chapter and Book gives each reader a sense of the importance of empathy. Not only is it crucial that we have compassion for others, we must also show compassion to ourselves.

I want to thank my family, friends, Resource Teachers and everyone who has helped me through showing and teaching me empathy throughout my life.

English Class

Elaine Feeney

1.

We decide to draw up class rules after arguing over,
We, Irish.
We decide the pronoun I is useful when speaking from memory.

I was alone in an mri scanner.
I was so filled with grief on a car journey from Syria to Lebanon
that I suffocated for a while in a tiny space beneath my siblings.

Class Note: I is often used by a nation's leader recounting success.
Eg. I opened a car factory. I will pay reparations.
But the class agree nations rely on they.

We decide the classroom needs better heating,
the hair-cut rule sucks
& some days are far worse days than other days.

Teacher Reflection in Margin:
I have developed a problem
teaching the collective We
E.g. We died in the famine (I did not)
E.g. We wrote in lyric poetry (The men)
E.g. We signed the Treaty (I did not)

Class Conclude:

We, Irish, is problematic to this class of Irish via England, English via Lagos, Lithuanian via New York to Ireland, Irish via Syria, Syrian-Irish via Lebanon & Greece & Waterford & Tuam, Polish via Russia, Irish via Poland, Irish Traveller via birth at halting site near Wembley Stadium.

2.

When summer comes, I say fresh cut grass is a cliché best avoided, the class says fresh cut grass brings holidays so We go outside and sit by the pitches. They describe the smell of a sweltering car, a burning building, honeysuckle, coconut sweets, sea spray that comes fast into a dinghy & what terror feels like in your nose.

Teacher Reflection in Margin:

have not experienced life as
a young boy who is now the man
of the house & no one knows
where his father is, no matter
how many times they ask.

They decide that it will be ok soon as summer is coming
& We agree that bad shit happens in the vacuous
space
created by power
& when anyone feels less than another
We agree the colour of the June sky is blue,
& sat on the grass,
We read aloud poems with no answers.

I Sure Hope the School around the Corner is Not the Same

Pat Dolan

Despite leading on a social research programme on the topic of empathy for many years now, it is somewhat ironic for me that my position and some of my core understanding of empathy and compassion still actually dates to my childhood and particularly to my school experiences. I was unfortunate and fortunate. Here is the unfortunate part. I was born the youngest of a large family in central Dublin and tragically my father died in a work accident when I was seven months old. This left my mother and older brothers and sisters having to cope with a major challenge. While attending a Christian Brothers school which overall was neither 'Christian or brotherly', I experienced and or witnessed violence and or emotional abuse, pretty much on a daily basis. Being left-handed did not help me either. It is my view, that the past excessive use of corporal punishment in Irish schools and the hurt and harm it caused, remains an unresolved issue for many of my generation and a remaining 'blot' on Ireland's social history. However, within this piece here I am not going to share the details of where and what I experienced or witnessed (that may be for another occasion). I am not willing to afford that space to the perpetrators who were both lay teachers and brothers. Suffice to say I remember them as adults out of any self-control who harmed children, sometimes for no apparent reason and often just deemed them to be disadvantaged, disabled or in some way different.

But here comes the fortunate component. Being resilient

in childhood to overcome adversity involves having protective factors in your life that can outweigh risk factors. Three protective factors were in place for me in school, without which frankly I would not have survived and thrived. Firstly, whereas I have no memory of my father, I was so fortunate in having a brilliant mother who compensated for this in so many ways and who ultimately epitomised to me what empathy is in real life. There is a difference between caring about another person and caring for another person – and she certainly cared for me. Not alone through her love did she let me know I was important, but she literally came to my school in my defence and 'took on' the perpetrators of violence and one lay teacher in particular – she could do social justice for sure!

Secondly, I was fortunate in that my older brothers and sisters cared as well. My brother Michael who is next in the family to me (we are Irish twins he is one year and a bit older than me) attended the same school at that time and had similar experiences. Not alone did he work to protect me and look out for me, but looking back, he did not just 'walk in my shoes' he 'walked with me in those shoes', and this helped me so much. Whereas like most young people we had friends in school, along with other peers who were cruel, Michael and I were (and still are) like 'two peas in a pod' as friends and brothers. We shared this solidarity despite the harming culture that the school allowed and even fostered. So, every day without fail, we left home together to walk to that school around the corner and waited for each other at the school gate at lunchtime and at closing time, to come home together – occasionally in silent and unspoken solidarity. Such was his support to me that when Michael finished school on completion of his leaving certificate, the loss of his company and support in part led to my somewhat premature departure from the school.

Thirdly and very importantly, I was also fortunate in that I learned quickly that not all the teachers were cruel, and some had humanity – there could be a light at the end of the tunnel. The one teacher who stands out for me, P.L., was like an oasis in a desert lacking humanity and warmth. He taught me English and apart from the fact that he was kind, and never resorted to violence or abusive behaviour with me or others in my class, he genuinely was interested in me and my learning. Two examples of his empathy and understanding remain with me. One of the 'fabled' offences we committed in school which frequently induced physical punishment was coming to school with long hair. Although this was fashionable in the early 1970s for some reason, still unknown to me to this day, it was deemed unacceptable behaviour. Whereas P.L. saw what was occurring and probably was restricted in what he could do about the rule and its brute force implementation by some brothers in particular, I remember him being interested in the fact that I was a Bob Dylan fan (something I garnered from my older brothers). He too was a Dylan fan and let me know that he thought Dylan's hair on the Blonde-on-Blonde album cover was really cool … this was his discrete way of protesting the crazy rule and showing some fellowship to me and others in the class. Similarly, around the same time, on one occasion when Michael and I were in Croke Park at a GAA match one summer Sunday afternoon, we happened to meet P.L. He showed us appropriate kindness through respectful recognition. He did not talk about school but was genuinely interested in our views of Dublin's performance on the day. These were two very simple yet effective acts of respect, which for me is the foundation of empathy.

So, in many ways because of the benefits of these supportive familial relationships in childhood and having at least one caring teacher in school, it is now somewhat easier for me to try to come to terms with and understand 'the others' not just as 'doers of evil' but as fellow humans with unresolved issues in their lives – why else would they have wanted to do such harm? I say this even if it is still difficult to forgive their behaviours. And I also say it knowing that no one is perfect all the time, including myself. As you will read from others in this book, it is really all about our collective understanding of empathy. Just as I am indebted to the other contributors in this book for increasing my learning, I also learn from my fellow editors. Mark (Brennan) in his essay has eloquently outlined a coping method to understanding the teachers who taught him, and Gillian (Browne) reminds me of the power of holding the positive esteem of another (her mother) as 'sailing high and salient', and Cillian (Murphy) who sets it out so simply for me. Empathy should be always active and not passive. As the late great Leonard Cohen reminds us 'There is a crack in everything, that is how the light gets in'.

Empathy in Education

Hugh Fitzmaurice

What is our intention currently in Irish Education?

What are we giving our attention to in our schools and colleges?

Is it people or processes? Is it outcomes or individuals?

Education comes from the Latin term *educere*, meaning 'to draw out'. What are we currently 'drawing out' from our youth and our educators? Are we creating reflective educational spaces where our inner horizons can flourish?

Imagine you are a student walking into an educational setting in 2021. You are aware that timetables, subjects, classrooms, exams, curricula, and discipline are all a priority. You know that schools are busy places where rules, expectations and judgements will be made day after day.

You know your efforts and outputs are assessed continuously. You know percentages, comments and reports are valued by teachers and parents. You know you will have assemblies or gatherings where you will be told how to behave and what to wear during your formative years.

Parent-teacher meetings are a commentary on your learning and educational experience but in most cases, you will not be present at these meetings.

You are aware that school never really ends at 4 o'clock because you know homework will be waiting. It is clear, consistent busyness is valued and cultivated in our schools.

These are all certainties in Education. These are the 'known knowns' as famously uttered by Donald Rumsfeld who once served as American Secretary of Defence. What are we modelling for the next generation?

What is unclear and uncertain is that YOU are valued, appreciated, and seen as an individual.

Are you ever asked how you are before you begin your learning just as a way of checking in?

Is school or college a space to reflect and grow emotionally and creatively? Can you express your vulnerability openly in an authentic safe space and feel heard and understood?

You may not know if your voice and your unique perspective will be deeply listened to and nurtured during your entire educational journey.

You may ask, when will the claws of constant striving, comparison and judgement release their grasp upon your young mind? You may wonder what is my value if I am not a certain percentage or academic ability?

What if the top priority in education was for you to be accepted for the gift of your beautiful uniqueness, your talents, your abilities, and insecurities?

When you entered the school gates aged four or five and you put your extraordinarily fragile and enthusiastic hand into your teachers' hand what did you hope for? What were your expectations and your wishes and wants?

Schools and colleges can often appear more interested in grading and defining who they assume you are rather than facilitating and supporting your evolving self.

I believe this paradigm needs a seismic shift and the priority needs to focus on creating space and time for students and their communities to reflect and really listen to each other.

It will make a big difference if time is allocated for each principal, teacher and student to be empathetically listened to without judgement in a safe space at different stages throughout every school week. This simple human act could create a sea-change in our experience of education in Ireland.

I believe it would really benefit our youth and our educators to share our common humanity and our authentic selves without fear and celebrate this in schools across this country. This is, 'drawing out' our humanity! This is 'gold' that we need to value more. This is putting the focus on connecting and understanding not comparing and competing.

This will help us further unlock fresh perspectives, new frontiers of thought and enhance the core of what schools are all about; Relationships with ourselves and others.

The poet and philosopher John Moriarty talked about the need to discover and see humanities 'sacred otherness'. He believed that when we make time and space and commit to asking, 'How are you', we could explore the world from new illuminating vantage points. He believed that taking this step with conviction is fundamentally more important than any exploratory mission into space, to the moon or Mars.

I believe it is now time in education to celebrate and connect with our common humanity, our interconnectedness. To explore new thresholds and frontiers of emotional growth, diverse intelligence, and a sense of human belonging by prioritising and activating Empathy in Education. When we feel more understood by our peers, studies show how this helps us to engage more, learn more and cultivate a sense of purpose in our lives.

We as schools and colleges can become Cathedrals of the Heart where young people's individuality matters.

Radical acts of reflection and action are needed now to ensure our humanity is central in education.

It is essential that Empathy in Education becomes as important and meaningful as Maths or English.

As an educator and parent, I believe Empathy in Education is not an add on. It is the heartbeat of who we are and needs to be a priority for our young people going forward. What we give our attention to now in our schools is the legacy we leave the next generation. Is Education to become a weapon of mass distraction or a space where the everyday micro moments of human connection, empathy and learning are valued and nurtured? We decide.

It's You I Like … The Way You Are Right Now

Dr Dana Winters and Dr Annie White

We begin all of our courses the same way. We ask each student to think about their own histories – who they are, who has loved them into being, what experiences have been instrumental to who they are in this moment. For some, this is a pleasant experience. For others, this can be painful and difficult. Understanding our histories is an important way of making sense of our present and planning for our futures. One course we offer is entitled 'What Would Fred Rogers Do?' Each year, 10–15 undergraduate students at Saint Vincent College, a small, Catholic, Benedictine, Liberal Arts College, enrol to learn more about Fred Rogers and think about how to extend his legacy in their own lives.

One semester, having asked students this same question about their own histories, a particularly tall young man finishing his final semester of college replied with a single statement: 'I am a jerk.' That was all he offered. I asked for more information, and he explained that everyone knows he's a jerk and that is who he is. There was pain in his face, hidden behind a superficial smirk and a football jersey.

During the course of the semester, we watched episodes of *Mister Rogers' Neighborhood*, listened to speeches offered by Fred Rogers, and read articles and letters written by Fred Rogers. As a class, we engaged with ideas such as compassion, difference, love, understanding and empathy. This same young man wrote papers relating his work as an Emergency Medical

Technician to his love of children and of helping others. He wrote about holding the hand of a young child after she had been in a car accident with her family; how he comforted her, distracted her and cared for her.

Fred Rogers was the creator and host of *Mister Rogers' Neighborhood*, which aired on public television from 1968–2001. For nearly 900 episodes, Fred invited children and families to be his 'neighbour', extending compassion and kindness into the homes of millions. In addition to that, Fred was a humanitarian, advocate and public intellectual. His archive currently boasts nearly 22,000 items, most of which are writings, original music compositions and correspondence.

At the Fred Rogers Institute we have the honour and responsibility of extending the legacy of children's television host Fred Rogers. Part of extending this legacy means introducing people to Fred for the first time. Most of our current students' lives no longer overlap with Fred Rogers, who died in February of 2003. It is sometimes hard for people to imagine a person who led with kindness and understanding, who focused on listening first and speaking second, who extended compassion for all people regardless of difference. This was Fred Rogers.

Though his television program was created for pre-school children, the messages he shared transcend childhood. As children, young people and adults, these messages continue to resonate many years later. Fred delivered his final commencement address in 2001 at Dartmouth College.[‡‡] Near the end of that speech, he recited the words from one of the songs he had written and composed for *Mister Rogers' Neighborhood*, entitled 'It's You I Like'. The words go like this ...

It's you I like,

‡‡ Rogers, F., (2002.) Dartmouth College 2002 Commencement Address. Accessed through Fred Rogers Archive, Latrobe, PA.

It's not the things you wear,
It's not the way you do your hair
But it's you I like
The way you are right now,
The way down deep inside you
Not the things that hide you,
Not your [caps and gowns]
They're just beside you.
But it's you I like
Every part of you.
Your skin, your eyes, your feelings
Whether old or new.
I hope that you'll remember
Even when you're feeling blue
That it's you I like,
It's you yourself
It's you.
It's you I like.

Having offered those lyrics, Fred followed up with an explanation of how they still apply to young people and adults, even 50+ years after he had written them for children. He said:

> And what that ultimately means, of course, is that you don't ever have to do anything sensational for people to love you. When I say it's you I like, I'm talking about that part of you that knows that life is far more than anything you can ever see, or hear, or touch. That deep part of you, that allows you to stand for those things, without which humankind cannot survive. Love that conquers hate. Peace that rises triumphant over war. And justice that proves more powerful than greed.
>
> So, in all that you do in all of your life, I wish you the strength and the grace to make those choices which will allow you and your neighbor to become the best of whoever you are.

Fred's words, messages and philosophies continue to resonate across time and space. He offers each of us a blueprint for understanding and empathy, if only we are willing to try. For our college students, Fred opens the door for each of them to be a person who extends care and kindness to others, even those who see themselves as someone very different.

When the course ended, the self-proclaimed 'jerk,' pulled me aside at his commencement ceremony. He hugged me and thanked me for exposing him to the ideas and teachings of Fred Rogers. I looked him in the eyes and told him he was not a jerk – he was so much more than what he thought he might be. He timidly agreed, and told me that, thanks to Fred Rogers, he saw that he was a helper, a care provider, and that he could be loved for those qualities. He could be liked. The way he is right now.

A Sheep among Wolves

Aisling Duffy

Knowing that we can be loved exactly as we are gives us all the best opportunity for growing into the healthiest of people – Fred Rogers

I wake up to the sound of light raindrops hitting the fogged up window, the sun hasn't risen yet so my shoe-box bedroom still feels cold and dark as it does during the night. My heart pounds as my mind becomes fully awake, I dread this feeling immensely, a sickness that consumes my body entirely, yet another day of feeling like a fish out of water. Eventually I soldier on and prepare myself quietly as usual, I tip toe down the stairs assuring I leave without encountering anyone. I stroll down the lonely street with my hood up, even though the rain has stopped, to keep myself invisible. I keep my head down and walk as slow as I possibly can to delay my arrival. As I reach the school gate the overwhelming feeling flows back in, I have to actively remind myself to breathe properly and push my body to move forward. I enter through the back, nobody comes in this way so I am safe to walk in without being noticed. I walk past a large group of girls who go silent once they spot me, they whisper as I pass, I could make out one of them saying 'she looks like a homeless woman' which is followed by a cluster of chuckles. I lock myself in one of the bathroom stalls and check my phone for the time, class starts in four minutes so I count down the seconds.

The day goes on as normal one class after the next the hours go by slowly, I keep to myself most of the time but occasionally glance and smile at someone that sits next to me, but I am usually met with an awkward look or slight scoff. I sit in the canteen during lunchtime, in the corner at a table that is majorly empty aside from one girl from a year below me that reads her book in solitude, I've never spoken to her, or her to me. We never have any food at home for lunch so I order soup and bread every day as it's the cheapest thing that's on offer. I distract myself on my phone and pretend like I'm elsewhere throughout all forty-five minutes. I get home by four o'clock and immediately try to sneak up to my room to avoid any confrontation, this time I'm unlucky and I run into my mother in the small front hallway. She looks at me as if I'm a stranger in her home, some intruder that has entered without knocking. 'Hello Emily I'm glad I caught you, I'm just going to ignore the fact that you've been avoiding me for the past few days' she obviously says this to attempt to make me feel bad, however I can't take her seriously as there is a massive food stain on her blouse that I just can't draw my attention away from. 'Your father is coming to see you this weekend with his new girlfriend, I'm hoping you can keep them happy by not moping around like you usually do, and if your father asks tell him I'm doing better than ever', she leaves the room in a calm anger, like she is trying to portray herself as completely unfazed yet I know that she is furious with just the mention of my father. As I meet my bedroom door my lungs become heavy, and my mind starts to run like a racehorse, I manage to lie on my back trying my best to breathe regularly. I remember reading in a self-help book about imagining a place to feel calm, so I close my eyes and force my imagination to work as hard as it can.

I enter a world that is filled with colour, at first glance it's a regular suburban neighbourhood with houses that line each side of the street, however when I look closer the houses become completely unique to those that sit next to them. Each house takes a different shape and size, and all of them are painted with different vivid colours, the street is symmetrically lined with trees that are fully flourished and flowers that are all in bloom, they almost look synthetic. The road that cuts this neighbourhood straight down the middle is smoothly paved, it looks and feels like a child's rendition of a town that was drawn with crayons and is proudly placed on the door of a fridge. I start to stroll down the empty street, there are cars parked in each driveway yet none exist on the road, it's almost completely silent except for the sound of birds chirping, their songs resemble a ringtone playing on repeat. My eyes start to adjust on a red trolley cart at the end of the street, it's stopped in its place as if it's waiting for me to board it, I hop on and it starts to move immediately. A man sits on the trolley behind me, I didn't notice him at first. I turn to look at him and he looks back at me with a warm welcoming smile, 'hello there, welcome to the neighbourhood' he exclaims excitedly, I felt extremely safe in his presence, even though this man was a complete stranger.

The cart enters through a dark tunnel but it exits through the other side before I can fear the darkness, the trolley stops at a beautiful garden with an arched entryway intertwined with vines and crimson red roses. The man jumps off the train, turns to me, and offers to show me around and with a pep in his step we wander into the park which is spectacularly decorated with thousands of flowers and plants. We pass a lady standing with a little boy, they both grin and wave at us as we walk by, and this same gesture is made by an older couple, all of them looking so happy and kind. We sit on a wooden bench which is placed next to a tall oak tree with dark green leaves.

The man asks me about myself, how is school, how is my mother, all questions that would be asked by someone I would know well or that would know me well. For some odd reason I am able to open up to him, I tell him that I don't have anyone to talk to and that my mother hasn't been very supportive since my dad left and that everyone around me treats me with contempt, I always feel like a sheep among wolves. He looks at me in a way that shows me that he is really listening, that he is taking in every single word that leaves my mouth. Once I stop talking, which feels like I've said everything I've ever wanted to say, the man says 'do you want to know what I think Emily?' he looks at me directly in the eyes and he takes a deep breath. 'I think that there is no person in the world like you, and I like you just the way you are' my eyes start to swell with tears as this man has just told me something that I haven't heard since I was a child, I can't remember ever feeling the way I feel having heard his words and how he made me feel by simply listening to me.

A clock tower rings somewhere in the distance and I realise that I'm running out of time, I must return to reality. I look at the man and thank him for listening and for being so understanding. 'Farewell neighbour' he responds quietly with the same smile that never left his face 'and always remember that you are not a sheep'. I board the cart once again and watch as the man waves goodbye, I close my eyes and feel the trolley move under the tunnel and when I open them I'm awake and in my bedroom.

It's morning again I must have fallen asleep, I'm still in my school uniform so I get up and brush myself off. Back to the real world I whisper to myself, I roll my eyes as my stomach sinks. I walk to school the same way I normally do, keeping my head down, I sit in my spot for lunch and notice the same girl sitting alone and reading her book, and the girl looks as isolated as I feel. I recall something the man on the trolley said to me 'if you could only sense how important you are to the lives of those you meet' so I build up the courage to sit closer to her, she looks up at me, I smile at her and she smiles back.

The Music Medicine Woman

Mary Coughlan

To be honest in the past I thought empathy was sympathy, and I didn't actually know the difference between the two. But through my life journey and as a result of my experiences good and bad, I am sure I know it now. Music has always been a core part of my life and in a good way. Many years ago I was really moved the first time I heard Christine McVie (Chicken Shack) sing so brilliantly *I'd Rather go Blind* by Ellington Jordan and Billy Foster. This was a song that really connected with my feelings and one that I went on to record and perform many times at gigs in Ireland and all around the world. At the time, while still very young I had separated from a boyfriend someone who was a little troubled as was I, and we had connected in our pain and the song held resonance for me. It still does. In many ways, it was the start of my realisation that music connects people emotionally.

Similarly at the age of seventeen on hearing Van Morrison sing *Listen to the Lion* the song affected me deeply and though I didn't know him, I felt he knew what I was going through … it was as if he was speaking to me personally. I did not realise it until much later that this was an 'anonymous' form of empathy.

So one of my key learnings in my career has been that singing connects people in terms of understanding each other. And, people who come to listen to me often connect very personally with the content and mood of the songs I sing. Indeed people have frequently written me notes during or after gigs saying that I am telling their story or that 'you know my life'. I really appreciate this when it happens and I like to think that at least some of the time my singing strikes a chord with people. They can understand the pain in the tone of my voice and they might just connect even from the mood of the music. I often sing of love, loss and pain and I think people identify with this. They can recognise it to the extent that even occasionally they may cry during a performance, which is great of course. Because I have seen this quite frequently and at gigs all over the world, it says to me that connection and compassion are a universal human response, regardless of who we were are or want to become.

In some cases, I have performed songs that people may not fully understand the details of and in countries far away from Ireland. However, they still connect deeply with the story of the song and show empathy for subjects. For example and in particular I recall singing the *Magdalene Laundry* in Australia and people I could see that the issue of stolen childhood and the type of pain the laundries brought about for young women and children and what horrors they endured was still recognised and respected.

In order to enable conditions for this expression through music for myself and others I use a breathing technique that opens up from deep inside me to the room for all and crucially is a safe and secure space. When this happens, I know it, I can feel it and there is a sense of great connection for me with the audience and I hope for them with me. It is empathy in action. It is a very powerful feeling. I am a medicine woman and music is my medicine.

In my life, I have enabled myself at a deep personal level to understand others which I suppose is core to being empathetic. In some ways, this has come about for me by dealing with my own past. But this was a hard journey for me. For example, as part of my shamanic training, I spent a day walking backwards in my grandmother's shoes in order to understand and make sense of my mother's life. I had to take this step backwards in order to forgive others and myself. I have learned that blaming is easy and compassion for self is really hard, but it is worth it, and I am still learning.

Nocturne II

John Kelly

I know when the fox is close –
the alarms of insomniac blackbirds
nesting foolishly under lights,
their heads turned by endless day.

Magpies too – all ratchety – and then
the yapping envy of domesticated dogs
tormented at windows and flaps – the old foxy stink
mocking what little they have left.

It's warm tonight, and not a breath. The universe
has me spotted, noted and forgotten about by now –
here in a busted armchair waiting for whatever comes:
vixen, hedgehog, leopard, ghost.

Grief, I tell myself, is never sadness unaccompanied.
In the apple tree I see an apple slowly turn,
unscrew itself and fall. It hits the ground
and lies there stunned – wondering what to do.

Savita

Inspiration Behind an Empathetic Revolution

Kitty Holland

The front page of *The Irish Times* the morning of Wednesday, 14 November 2012 shocked the world, convulsed Ireland and began an 'empathetic revolution' for Irish women and girls.

Dominated by the radiant face of a young Indian woman, resplendent in her traditional dress for the Diwali festival the previous month, it was accompanied by the headline: 'Woman, "denied a termination" dies in hospital.'

It went on to tell how just three weeks earlier, Savita Halappanavar (31), a dentist, had presented with back pain at Galway University hospital, had been found to be miscarrying, and had died of septicaemia a week later.

The article, written by me and my colleague Paul Cullen, continued: 'Her husband, Praveen Halappanavar (34), an engineer at Boston Scientific in Galway, says she asked several times over a three-day period that the pregnancy be terminated. He says that, having been told she was miscarrying, and after one day in severe pain, Ms Halappanavar asked for a medical termination.

'This was refused, he says, because the foetal heartbeat was still present and they were told, "this is a Catholic country".

'She spent a further 2½ days "in agony" until the foetal heartbeat stopped.

'The dead foetus was removed and Savita was taken to the high dependency unit and then the intensive care unit, where she died of septicaemia on the 28th of October.

'Speaking from Belgaum in the Karnataka region of south-west India, Mr Halappanavar said an internal examination was performed when she first presented.

'The doctor told us the cervix was fully dilated, amniotic fluid was leaking and unfortunately the baby wouldn't survive.' The doctor, he says, said it should be over in a few hours. There followed three days, he says, of the foetal heartbeat being checked several times a day.

'Savita was really in agony. She was very upset, but she accepted she was losing the baby. When the consultant came on the ward rounds on Monday morning Savita asked if they could not save the baby, could they induce to end the pregnancy. The consultant said, 'As long as there is a foetal heartbeat we can't do anything'.

'Again on Tuesday morning, the ward rounds and the same discussion. The consultant said it was the law, that this is a Catholic country. Savita [a Hindu] said: 'I am neither Irish nor Catholic' but they said there was nothing they could do.

'That evening she developed shakes and shivering and she was vomiting. She went to use the toilet and she collapsed. There were big alarms and a doctor took bloods and started her on antibiotics.

'The next morning I said she was so sick and asked again that they just end it, but they said they couldn't.'

At lunchtime, the foetal heart had stopped and Ms Halappanavar was brought to theatre to have the womb contents removed. 'When she came out she was talking okay but she was very sick. That's the last time I spoke to her.'

At 11 p.m., he got a call from the hospital. 'They said they were shifting her to intensive care. Her heart and pulse were low, her temperature was high. She was sedated and critical but stable. She stayed stable on Friday but by 7 p.m. on Saturday, they said her heart, kidneys and liver weren't functioning. She was critically ill. That night, we lost her.'

Savita had died at 1.09 a.m., Sunday, 28 October 2012.

Calls from Irish news outlets, seeking interviews about the story, started coming from 6 a.m. the morning of publication. The first was from Newstalk radio, quickly followed by RTÉ's morning radio-news programme, Morning Ireland. Then Today FM, Galway Bay FM, Highland Radio, TV3, UTV and BBC Northern Ireland.

The death of a young, healthy woman, with the added dimension that she had sought an abortion which her family argued would have saved her life, was a huge Irish story.

Unexpected, by me anyway, were the calls that soon poured in from international news outlets – CNN, the BBC World Service, Channel 4 News, Sky News, Al Jazeera, France 24, El Pais. Later, as dawn broke across the Atlantic, calls started from the *New York Times,* the *Washington Post,* CNN.

The one news outlet Praveen, who was still in India, agreed I could share his number there with was RTÉ. That lunchtime he spoke to broadcaster Sean O'Rourke, on the *News at One.* Toward the end of the almost ten-minute interview, he recounted Savita's last minutes.

> That night [early Sunday 28 October] at around one o'clock the nurse came running. I was just standing outside the ICU. She, she just told me to pray and she took me near Savita and she said: 'Will you be OK to be there during her last few minutes?' I said, 'Yes I want to'. I was holding her hand. They were trying to pump her heart. There was a big team around her and the doctor just told me, they just lost her.

Orla O'Connor, chief executive of the National Women's Council told me after: 'Praveen changed everything. He was so clear and so public and so powerful. He said they had requested an abortion, and she had died. That affected a lot of men as well as women.'

That evening, in response first to a Facebook post calling for a protest outside the Dáil, a call repeated across social media, thousands gathered outside Leinster House. In the dark, cold November evening they carried candles and held placards with such slogans as, 'I have a heartbeat too' and 'I am here to apologise for my country'.

Sinead Kennedy, abortion rights activist who had put up the initial Facebook post and MC'd the vigil recalls: 'It was very quiet. People were crying. People were holding candles, pictures of Savita. It had a really sombre, sad, shocked tone. It felt almost like being at a funeral.

'There were just so many people there who I think had had no intention of going to a rally that evening but had gone, on their way home, just to be there ... Everyone was just very aware it was important to be there and I think people felt that weight of responsibility.'

That vigil, and many more like it across Ireland, began in earnest a campaign to repeal the 8th amendment from the Irish Constitution, a campaign that would won by a margin of 66.4 per cent six years later.

The eighth amendment to *Bunreacht na hÉireann* was made in 1983, when Article 40.3.3 was inserted into it following a bitterly divisive referendum campaign.

The pro-amendment arguments had won on 7 September that year, by a margin of 66.9 per cent.

Article 40.3.3 provided an equal right to life to the unborn child and to the mother carrying it – effectively banning abortion in all circumstances. It said: 'The State acknowledges the right to life of the unborn and, with due regard to the equal right to life of the mother, guarantees in its laws to respect, and, as far as practicable, by its laws to defend and vindicate that right'.

While it was, and by many continues to be, portrayed as a caring and empathetic Article, it effectively diminished what Praveen in one interview had described as 'the bigger life' – i.e. the mother's.

It meant the unborn's life had to be protected just as much as the mother's life in all circumstances. And it certainly had to be protected more than the mother's health, mental well-being, never mind her hopes and dreams, even in such circumstances as rape and incest.

It gave rise to a huge export market in crisis pregnancies as women (who could afford to) travelled in their thousands every year to Britain for abortions.

It also resulted in myriad crisis cases, several of which ended up before the Irish courts as lawyers (most of them men) argued before judges (most of them men) as to whether or not the woman or girl who was the subject of their particular proceedings should be allowed have an abortion in Ireland, or indeed even be allowed travel for an abortion.

In all of these the women or girls remained anonymous, given only alphabet letters to identify them. Each is worth looking up if you are interested. They are: the 'X' case (1992); the 'C' case (1997); 'D' v Ireland at the European Court of Human Rights (ECHR) (2005); Miss 'D' (2007), and, 'A', 'B' and 'C' v Ireland at the ECHR (2010).

Each brought pro-choice and anti-abortion protestors onto the streets. Each dominated media agendas for days and weeks. Each led to hand-wringing and political commitments to address the abortion dilemma.

None, however, had the impact Savita had. While the cases of the previous two decades had elicited people's anger, sadness and empathy, the empathy had no 'target', no knowable woman or girl with whom to connect.

In Savita, however, we had not only her name, but her face too. And in Praveen we had a calm, dignified and resolute voice for her truth – a voice that could not but demand our empathy. And that was transformative.

Within an hour of Praveen speaking on radio that Wednesday lunchtime, women, more and more of them, were speaking their truth. Directly after the lunchtime news, RTÉ radio's popular, daily phone-in show, *Liveline*, was dominated by women telling their stories of having been denied abortions, or of having had difficult miscarriages in Irish hospitals. Their calls filled the programme for the following two days, as women – many of them giving their own names – spoke publicly about crisis pregnancies in a way not heard on Irish broadcast media before.

They described the isolation, shame, fear and pain they had felt, and the near total absence of support they had in Ireland.

One, who gave the name Carolyn, had experienced a trauma strikingly similar to that of Savita, twenty-seven years previously. At sixteen weeks' pregnant she was having her third miscarriage. When she presented as a hospital a foetal heartbeat was detected.

'It was made clear to me that nothing could be done until I was seen by a gynaecologist. I tried to tell them what needed to be done. I was in extreme pain, much more than in my first and second miscarriages. I did try to say what was needed now was a D and C [dilation and curettage]. I had had one at my first and second miscarriages which took place in London. I was told I would have to wait.

'I was brought to a ward and I remember it was the first time in my life when really I had lost control. I was in so much pain I was wailing and terribly distressed. I think I asked for pain relief and I was told it couldn't be administered because of the fact there was a baby.

'While I was lying there the hard, cold reality of my situation dawned on me. It was the mid-1980s and the Society for the Protection of the Unborn Child was quite prominent and it just dawned on me that this was probably down to me or the baby. I realised very clearly that I might die and that was what I felt more than anything. The fear was indescribable – that I might die.'

Her gynaecologist arrived some hours later and performed a D and C.

'He saved my life and I was enormously grateful,' said Carolyn. 'When I woke up this morning and heard this news of this girl in Galway the thought that crossed my mind was that twenty-seven years later this kind of thing could actually still happen. I had clearly believed that in the interim more enlightened legislation [was in place].'

Carolyn's was among the first of thousands of women who, between then and May 2018 when the 8th was repealed, would tell their stories, finding empathetic listeners and solidarity in each other and from everyone who cared about them. Their voices transformed the narrative.

As they told their stories, other women, including often much older women, found their voices. They told stories over the next six years, not just about abortion, but about miscarriage, about not being told why their babies had died in birth, or had been born with severe disabilities, about sustaining life-changing injuries during child-birth and not being told why; about not being able to conceive – about not being listened to, heard or taken seriously. And about shame, they refused to hold as theirs any longer.

The discussion became no longer just about the rights of

the unborn, but also and even more so about the lived realities of Irish women and girls. The nucleus around which this transformation happened was the heartfelt, anguished, grieving, angry, loving and growing empathy for the too-often, silent pain endured by too many of our women and girls.

Savita, without a doubt, started the empathetic revolution that changed Ireland for women and girls. Her enduring centrality was clear the sunny, Saturday morning of 26 May 2018 that followed a day of jubilation at the referendum result.

At a mural – a reproduction of the image of Savita used six years earlier on the front of *The Irish Times* – by the Aches graffiti artists in the Portobello area of Dublin, people gathered to reflect, weep, lay flowers and leave notes of sorrow and gratitude.

'I voted for you Savita. May you rest in peace. You'll never be forgotten along with all the other women who suffered. All my love xxx', said one.

'Sorry, really sorry', said another, while one woman wrote: 'It is the biggest shame that your death galvanised repeal of our 8th Amendment that failed you. I'm so sorry Savita. Love Annie.'

More briefly, but speaking for many hundreds of thousands whose votes were born of true empathy, another said: 'Sorry we were too late but we're here now. We didn't forget about you'.

Lonely Hearths

Gillian Browne

Her seat, kept warm beside the fire
Sits empty now
The memory of her strong

The universal pathos of grief
To walk in another's shoes
Family, friends the community
They understand the assignment

Home-cooked dinners
Salad sandwiches
Scones
Stories shared remembering how lucky we were
All magically appear

This coat of grief wears heavy
Bearing it made easier
By others, my empaths
Helping carry the weight

Empathy for My Mother

Dermot Whelan

'I know it. I know they're taking my things.'

We're side by side on your couch. My hand rests on yours.

'Let's breathe,' I say. You try but your breath is anxious and shallow.

'That's not my chair. I want my chair.'

Your eyes search the room for reassurance. Your grip tightens.

'Let's keep breathing. That's it. Into your belly.'

Strangeness seeps into your view like dusk. I try to imagine what it's like. I get flashes. I think I know but it's fleeting.

You're so worried. And my heart breaks. I can't reach you. It's a conversation in a howling gale. Helplessness is a sea. Shore long forgotten.

'These are all your things, Mum. You just have difficulty remembering them because your brain isn't working properly.' It sounds clunky and childish and harsh.

There is a flash of quiet understanding on your face. Then the anxiety returns. Your eyes dart once more and the breath quickens.

'Let's do our breathing. Slow, deep breath into the belly. Gentle breaths out. That's it.'

Your hand is warm.

So much has disappeared. So much has faded. So much has dissolved.

But not your breath. It remembers everything.

The Magic Cauldron

Susan McKeown

In 2013, I brought my then ten-year-old daughter back to Ireland from Manhattan to live for a while. It wasn't something she thanked me for at the time, but I was after something and this was the only way I could think of to get it. I wanted her to have an experience beyond being able to say 'my mom's Irish': I wanted her to know what it was like to grow up in Ireland. I've always told her it's a mix, that many of us have a love-hate relationship with what it means to be Irish: there are parts of being Irish I'm always deeply connected to, and parts I've often felt isolated from. In some way, I hoped to be part of finding new ways of healing for ourselves and future generations, and I knew I needed to start by learning about the ways I needed to heal myself.

There were other factors too. In the years before, the restructuring of the music industry caused by Spotify meant that little was left for the actual creators of the music and so, like many songwriters I had to look for new ways to support myself and my daughter. I produced community culture and mental health projects in the US and Ireland that were featured on national public radio and then one day I heard the computer scientist Jaron Lanier on the radio articulating, as few others have, the detrimental impact that capitalism and 'disruptive technologies' were having on society and I made up my mind to go back. The quote that stuck in my mind was 'young people today have a reduced expectation of what a person is, and who they can become'. It reminded me of something I once read from our great social historian Joe Lee about how the impact of colonialism shrivelled Irish perspectives on Irish potential.

In Dublin, I enrolled my daughter in fifth class and myself in business school. When I graduated I spent three years doing research and development: facilitating projects with youth in Ireland and New York, many living with economic deprivation, in public housing, in direct provision, in the traveller community. I had lost my savings producing a hugely ambitious New York Irish cultural festival in twenty-six venues in 2016 so I had no choice but to go slow and steady. When it was sometimes difficult, I reminded myself that I had asked for this, that I was getting what I asked for, and that this was how it felt.

In the old annals it is written that the first people who came to Ireland were 'a dark race who came from the four corners of the sky' and brought with them four sacred tools of power. One of these was a magic cauldron from which no one who ate went away unsatisfied, and in some stories had the power to bring the dead back to life. This story was the focus for a project our organisation produced with youth living in direct provision in St Patrick's Accommodation Centre in Monaghan in 2018. We visited the Monaghan County Museum to see the splendid cauldrons in its collection, and it was easy to imagine their contents satisfying the hunger of entire communities in Ireland long ago, as well as restoring to health strangers who were hungry and worn out from journeying.

When I landed as an immigrant on the Lower East Side, I had no idea I would spend my adult life there. It was an amazing place for musicians when there was a music scene, before all the clubs disappeared, before the artists moved away because they could no longer afford to live there, before the small stores closed down and Target, 7-Eleven and Trader Joe's moved in. The Cuala Foundation develops cultural projects that connect youth more deeply with themselves and their community and we recently partnered with Amerinda (American Indians Artists, Inc.) for a proposal to restore and reclaim an abandoned bathhouse as a community cultural hub. We worked together envisioning a space for community knowledge and practice, where older teens and young adults will have time and space to make art, and earn incentives for participating in community projects, and where our Native American brothers and sisters who have been there all along can teach us about the indigenous ways of the land to which we all now belong, so that we can better understand how to take care of it and each other.

It's critical for youth to know community history, the struggles the people have faced and the ways they have resisted and survived. The societal problems we're dealing with today took root long ago and are very entrenched: many times I heard the expression 'Ireland doesn't like change'. We still have the highest rates in Europe of suicide for young women and girls and among the highest for young men and boys. My friend Will Hall is a survivor of suicide and a mental health counsellor. He says suicidal feelings often aren't giving up on life, but instead a conflict between wanting to change your life and not feeling any power to make change – and the key becomes finding that power. I can understand people thinking that nothing would ever change in the Ireland in which I grew up. Younger generations might find it hard to believe how we accepted the injustice of the systems that dominated, but for most of us the options were few, the traditional one being emigration.

It's not the people who are broken but the systems in which we are living, where value is falsely attributed to wealth and status. These addictive systems keep us distracted and isolated and deny the value inherent in each human life, and that in healthy, whole communities every voice is important and needed. Belonging is a process that moves at the speed of trust, a call and response like a traditional song that goes back and forth between singers and never really ends, each singer bringing their own voice and expression to the whole and finding its place to belong. I'm very conscious of those who left Ireland before me and the reasons why they did. Some never come back, like the hundreds of thousands of young women who travelled alone to America in the nineteenth century and never returned. But I came home. I was warned that re-entry could be bumpy – and it was – but I'm grateful for the individuals and community groups who have welcomed and accepted me and taught me so much about the value of what it means to be Irish and what it means to belong.

Does it Count as Empathy if You Learn it the Hard Way?

Brendan O'Connor

I'm not sure. Does it count as empathy if you learn it the hard way? Is there anything noble in gaining an understanding of other people's lives only because your own life becomes another person's life? Is that empathy? Or is that cheating?

I made it through school without knowing anyone gay. Strange isn't it? That out of the hundreds of guys (only guys) I came up with, not one of them was gay. There were no gay guys, just some guys who were accused of being 'benders', as banter. Quiet guys often. That was what passed for harmless fun back then.

But it would be college before I met anyone who was gay.

Now, I can imagine what it must have been like for some of those guys in school, where nobody was gay. Not one.

I knew one guy who was Egyptian. One brown guy. There was nobody black. Nobody in school, nobody in the area. We grew up with people like us. And we just assumed everyone was like us. Maybe there were gay people and black people in Dublin.

I didn't know anyone with a disability either. I saw them all right. I saw the odd person with Down syndrome, around the place with their parents, who seemed older than the rest of our parents. And when we would go swimming in Lota, sometimes you might catch a glimpse of one of the residents, maybe behind a window, locked away in their world.

At Christmas Joan Murphy would bring us out to the Cork

Spastic Clinic for a concert. Joan Murphy was one of those women who might not have talked much about empathy, but who had a heart as big as Ireland, and who bled what we now know as empathy all over every situation she went into. Joan taught me piano and singing and elocution. But Joan also taught me other things. Like when we went to the Spastic Clinic, and we were as terrified of the kids there as they were of us. Joan treated them just like she treated us, and spoke to them as if they were just like us, and laughed with them, and showered them with warmth, as if they were just like us, and was stern with them sometimes too, as if they were just like us.

I never really cracked the piano, and it took a long time for some of Joan's other lessons to sink in.

I feel ashamed to say this now, but when my daughter Mary was born with Down syndrome, I knew my life was ruined. I remember I rang my brother in America and told him. My life is ruined.

It's imprinted on me, the slow emotion replay of that day, as the mood changed in the operating theatre where the caesarean was being done. She came out not floppy, which is what you want. But then they brought her over to the table, and started looking at her, and talking amongst themselves, and suddenly the colour drains out of everything. And when the doctor said Trisomy 21 to us, in heavily accented English, we didn't know what he was talking about.

And then it became clear, but I knew this couldn't be happening, because this was the kind of thing that happened to other people. These things did not happen to people like us. That sounds harsh. But that was how it seemed back then, because back then I knew nothing.

And since then, I have lived someone else's life. And maybe in some ways it's a harder life, but it's also a better life. And now I understand so much more. And now, when I see people who look pityingly at us, the way I might have looked pityingly at a family like ours before, I try to be kind, because I know they know nothing. I can tell they think that it's nice that we are doing our best, with the cross we have to bear in life, but that really we are just pretending. They think we are just trying to get on with it. They also often think that we are good people, more saintly, more patient.

We are not. But we think we know things they don't know. Because we think we know a different kind of love, a love that most of them will never know. It can be a challenging kind of love, but that only serves to make it a more practical, muscular kind of love. It's not always fluffy. Maybe it's love as it should be, hard work sometimes.

We think we have a clarity that lots of those people will never have. I think I know what true unconditional love is. I know love that forces you to go to war for the loved one.

I love smart people, but I don't tend to judge people too much based on their intelligence – though maybe on their ignorance. I am free from worrying what my kids will achieve on any conventional metric. I know that the only thing that matters is that they are happy.

If I had known my daughter forty years ago, I might have been afraid of her, if indeed I ever even came across her. I might have seen her through a window when I went swimming, locked in that other depressing world that people like her inhabited, that smelled like hospital, and that looked like the beige of institutions.

She has given me many gifts. But perhaps the most important one is that my definition of people like me has broadened, and I meet them all where they are, looking neither up nor down, nor awkwardly at them. The broken people are my people too now, and the ones who have fixed themselves and come out the other side more interesting and open, and the mad ones, and the ones who don't fit in, and the ones who struggle, and the ones who have had to learn unlimited love, the ones who are challenged, who don't get given a chance, who are happy despite not having what we are taught is the right kind of life, the ones who have to fight, the self-pitying ones, the self-destructive ones.

And it's not quite empathy, and it's slightly cheating, and I don't always manage to practise it, and I'm challenged every day by it. But the best we can all do is to try to understand that our common humanity doesn't reside in perfection. It's in our faults, and our failings, and our shocks and the mishaps that nearly break us, and in our weaknesses that demand of us more courage, and in our shame and our difference. And maybe the best we can do is try to look across at each other at the same level and silently acknowledge, while we are all fucked up in different ways, and while we all have different stuff, and some of us have better luck and some of us have worse luck, we are all brothers and sisters in our common fuckedupness.

So we don't need to feel sorry for each other. We just need to remember that we all have our story that got us to here, and I could be you if I had your bad luck or good luck. And you could be me.

Hot Wheels, Warm Heart

Tara Dawson

Growing up I always thought of myself as a sensitive child, who was strongly affected by the emotions of those around me, both highs and lows. Throughout my life, I have always viewed this as a negative trait, believing I needed to toughen up and not let myself become so affected by the feelings of others. However, now as a young adult, I have come to realise that this is simply empathy and it is one of my biggest strengths. It helps me to understand the emotions of others and recognise their feelings, providing me with the opportunity to build lifelong social connections based on compassion and kindness.

I have learned that just because you don't agree with somebody it doesn't mean you can't empathise with them. This isn't sympathising with someone from a distance, but instead truly realising the depth of their emotions and being able to actively feel for this person rather than simply feeling sorry for them. I have learned that in certain situations you have to be able to put aside your feelings of what you believe is 'right or wrong', eliminating all judgement and instead embrace the emotions of others.

I believe that my empathetic nature has developed due to growing up with a disabled parent, whose condition has progressed throughout my life. Consequently, this empathy developed concurrently with the challenges my dad encountered as time passed by. Growing up as a child with a disabled parent is an entirely unique experience that comes with a number of struggles and negative realities. It forced me to grow up quicker than an average child would and took away a number of childhood experiences, such as, riding a bike with my dad, having a father-daughter dance and playing games outside together. Despite this, my dad has always taught me to appreciate the things that we can do together rather than dwell on the things that we can't, such as sitting on my dad's lap while he drives around the house in his electric chair, laughing and swinging across the bedroom in his hoist, decorating his wheelchair with lights and tinsel at Christmas. Being brought up to appreciate these things in life and be kind to those who are struggling has made me the empathetic individual I am today.

In addition to my personal journey of empathy, the small community I come from in Donegal has been nothing but empathetic, generous, and compassionate towards my family. My dad suffers from secondary progressive Multiple Sclerosis (MS) and in 2017, as a family we came to the harsh reality that my dad was beginning to lose his battle, so we decided to take the risk of sending my dad to India to receive potentially life-changing stem cell treatment. This treatment came with a huge risk factor as it is known to be the most aggressive form of stem cell treatment with high percentages of people not making it through the process, however, if it was to work it is the most effective form of treatment and could change my dad and family's life forever. To send my dad to India this was going to cost us €32,000 which as a family we could simply not afford, therefore we decided to reach out to our community for some help. We did this by setting up a GoFundMe page, bucket collecting and organising fundraising events such as coffee mornings, raffles, dinner dances and 10k walks.

Not only did endless individuals generously donate money through our fundraising page, but we had a number of local businesses offering their time, money, and even to host events so that we could reach our end goal. We had local pubs hosting quiz nights, local PTs hosting exercise classes, a 'Come Dine with Me' held by the local GAA club, a 10k sponsored walk and a charity cycle & run, to name a few. We also held a silent auction where all the prizes were kindly donated, such as a trip for two to Celtic Park (including coach, ferry and match tickets), autographed sports jerseys, and vouchers from local salons and makeup artists. The level of generosity and understanding shown within our community was astounding, and we are forever grateful for the degree of compassion that was shown. Each individual who donated and assisted us in our journey demonstrated their ability to understand and actively feel what we were going through as a family, and if it wasn't for this ability to empathise then we would not be where we are today, and I am eternally grateful for this.

Empathy is a precious trait to have; it has helped me to view the world in a more understanding and balanced way, increasing the level of positivity in my life and in the lives of those around me. I have realised that in a way empathy is contagious, when you actively show understanding towards an individual they will reciprocate this feeling and carry it with them throughout their life. Therefore, if we all make a conscious effort to empathise with those around us rather than sympathising from a distance, the world will become a better place full of balance and appreciation, and to me that is a beautiful world worth living in.

Empathy as an Act of Defiance

The Edge

So why are humans sensitive to the emotional state of others? The answer might not be very romantic but evolution seems to have bequeathed us this ability because it conveys an advantage; cementing social cohesion and allowing us to build family groups and communities. But just in case our instinct for fellow-feeling gives us a collective swelled-head, it should be pointed out that other species have the ability to feel empathy. As well as all higher primates, dogs, mice, elephants and rats also look out for their friends.

If we are not unique in having this ability, we may be unique in suffering its absence. The inability to empathise is a tell tale sign of mental illness. Few of us could imagine being callous enough to seriously injure or kill someone else with emotional impunity. We use words to describe those who can with a degree of reassuring separation: 'Psychos', 'Monsters', 'Sickos'. Empathy relies on a degree of commonality and is therefore reserved for people like us; those who think like us, speak like us, and to put very basically could be us. We empathise when we can relate.

Those others, who are different to us, are excluded because we don't know what they are about. They might be a threat. They might be about to steal our food, our parking spot, our girlfriend, our job. They inspire fear. There are endless ways and justifications that we use to 'other' people. It is another evolutionary survival adaptation. There are times when we absolutely need to protect ourselves from aggression or malevolent intent. There is however this grey area of risk that is really only a perception. Most of the time, we get to decide. It's a choice, a habit, a state of mind, a philosophy. Right now in our ultra-sophisticated global society, equipped with instant access to boundless amounts of information, of varying qualities, we are regressing into a pre-enlightenment tribalism. Fear has been weaponised by deeply cynical politicians who play us and our fears like violins. Barriers based on belief and identity are turning our society into an array of ideological ghettos. Mistrust and paranoia are at an all-time high. We are in serious danger of unleashing psychopathic tendencies on a societal level. We have seen this movie before. It doesn't end well. So what to do?

Empathy involves a decision and for it to mean anything, it should accommodate the potential for change. A change of understanding. The genuine attempt to understand and put yourself in the shoes of someone who is not like you, does not speak like you, think like you and therefore could not be you, is horizon expanding. Those 'others', of whatever kind, are worthy of our empathy not just because we might learn how to accept them as one of us, but because in the process of opening up to them they might just be inspired to do the same for you or me, or some other of their 'others'. Daryl Davis, the black musician who has converted Ku Klux Klan members by simply sitting down and talking to them, is a great example. At times like this, and particularly at the flash points of society, the decision to empathise is an act of defiance against the prevailing trend. An enlarged empathy might just be our saving grace.

Empathy, the Best Superpower

Rabbi Zalman Lent

His name is Ibere Ugochukwu, he is a street vendor in Lagos, Nigeria, and whenever he sees a prison truck transporting new prisoners, he rushes over and pushes food through the bars, free of charge. Why does he do that?

A number of years ago I was becoming disillusioned as the internet seemed to slowly transform from the source of all types of information and communication to the source of all types of hatred and intolerance. It seemed to get worse day-by-day as the anonymity it provided allowed people to show their darker sides. Students I knew were being harassed online and I had simply stopped reading the comments on articles of interest as they were often so filled with vitriol and abuse.

That is when I saw the story of Ibere Ugochukwu, arrested and violently tortured after being falsely accused of theft from his place of employment in Lagos, Nigeria. It was on a site called Humans of New York (HONY) and there was a photograph of Ibere with boxes of food balanced on his head. After his awful experience as a prisoner deprived of food, once released he decided to hawk food near the prison, so that as the prison trucks drove by he would be able to give the new inmates some food – he used his great suffering as a catalyst to do greater good.

As I was reading that story I broke my habit and glanced at the comments, which I was pleasantly surprised to find were all positive; none of the usual racism, slurs and hatred, just an outpouring of empathy, love, care and generosity. People were inspired, they wanted to help, to support, to show kindness.

Humans of New York is what I like to call the kind corner of the internet, a safe place to read about the struggles and traumas others are going through and to then see them virtually embraced by the thousands of messages of support. It is a rare find, a popular website read by many millions where it is hard to find a note of negativity. There are many stories of loss and pain, and even of torture and suffering, but all are inspirational in that often they have an inspiring ending as people rose to meet their challenges, but even if not, the immediate feedback is inspirational in and of itself. Myriads of readers from a panoply of backgrounds, colours, creeds and cultures all sending their love and kindness in a surge of empathy that is hard to find anywhere else outside special interest or support groups.

If only we could clone that model onto more parts of the internet, what a great society we would be. A society where every individual feels listened to, validated, cared for and supported with respect and empathy. Currently that is not the case, and the statistics about the negative effects of social media platforms are terrifying. The flood of abuse and epithets showered upon anyone slightly different, or with an alternative opinion are simply awful, and a serious contributing factor to the poor self-image of many in society, especially young teens.

It needs to change.

Kindness and compassion are cornerstones of Judaism; so much so that we are told to question the lineage of someone cruel or callous – do they really belong as part of our people? This need for kindness is not just an abstract ideal, this is embedded in Jewish law, based on the frequent Torah verses encouraging empathy – cautioning us to care for the widow and the orphan, to give tithes for the poor and to pay wages on time, to care for the sick and respect the elderly. It extends to animals too – to help unload a fallen pack-animal, even if it belongs to an enemy; to shoo away the mother bird before taking her eggs and so on. These are not just Jewish laws, they are humane values for all of God's children – to constantly be cognisant of another's feelings, and do our best to help where possible, or at the very least not to be 'a stumbling block for the blind' in any way, shape or form.

What is refreshing about HONY, and its creator Brandon Stanton, is that he finds – amongst the anguish – so many moments of beauty, enough to give us hope that the world is not devoid of love or empathy. In one moving vignette, he interiews a Russian orphan abandoned at a young age by an alcoholic father. The young man credits his then teacher in the orphanage, Anna Mihailovna, with never giving up on him, constantly pushing him to succeed, and encouraging him to try to get adopted. In a moving twist to the story, he did find a potential adoptive family who even flew him out to Italy to visit, but on his return to Russia he lost their information and was unable to contact them. Fifteen years later, he found the slip of paper with their contact details by chance, and made the call. Amazingly, they still remembered him and repeated their offer of adoption which he accepted, giving him a new lease of life and potential.

The world is full of good people like Ibere Ugochukwu, Anna Mihailovna and the adoptive family from Italy, but we tend not to highlight them as it doesn't make for such interesting headlines. Maybe all we really need to do is to put stories like that on the front pages and in the headlines and move the murderers and evildoers to the footnotes? If only it were that simple. Yet, each of us in our own lives can indeed do good, we can really be agents for positive change, by doing acts of goodness and kindness.

My late teacher and spiritual guide, Rabbi Schneerson zt'l,

known as the Rebbe of Lubavitch, was once visited by a group of disabled army veterans to receive his blessing. One of the group had lost mobility due to injury and was confined to a wheelchair. He felt bitter and angry about his injuries and even his close friends had difficulty discussing it with him. After the Rebbe's address and blessing, he came over to each of the soldiers and spoke a few words, but to this wheelchair-bound young man, he simply looked deeply into his eyes and said, 'Thank You'.

With those two words, said with deepest empathy and understanding, the young man felt a great sense of freedom, as his bitterness and anger at the world dissipated. Sometimes that is all it takes.

Our words and actions hold immense power, both the things we do and say and those we hold back from doing or saying. Using the innate power we possess to make someone else's life brighter can have a ripple effect with far-reaching consequences, gradually making the world a happier, more caring and more empathetic home for us all; let's not waste any time.

My Power Called Empathy

Matthew Shaw-Torkzadeh

I think to myself wow, I must have powers to feel your pain
although it is just a skill I've learned and trained.
Your eyes wide open you must be in disbelief,
You're angry I can see when you clench your teeth.
I look at my surroundings and see a boy about to take the final shot to win the match
and I use my power to visualise his pressure,
the ref then proclaims that they have lost the game.
I open my eyes and see his sorrow as he has missed the shot,
I look at a tear in his eye as he breaks down and starts to cry.
My superpower couldn't have done anything to help,
But that feeling,
I really felt.

The next day I was walking along
I saw another boy standing alone.
His hands shaking a tear in on his cheek,
He was holding a sheet of paper
He was about to freak.
I saw that it was a test
One he hadn't done well on,
But tried his very best.
He was so upset he that he could only focus on that paper as if everything around him has gone.
I could tell it was an important one,

I used my power to feel his stress
That pain like a press in the middle of your chest.
As he walked away my power helped me realise he
wanted to be left alone,
He tried to not draw attention by texting on his phone.
But I know sooner or later he will need to talk.
I realise now whenever you feel like the only one in pain,
Know there is someone who feels the same.
Or maybe might understand and give you a helping
hand.

Empathy as a Broader Understanding of Family

Valerie Biden Owens

In late August 2020, my brother accepted the Democratic Party's nomination for President of the United States. In his speech that night, he talked about the global pandemic we were experiencing and the resulting economic crisis it had caused, two things that were on the minds of all Americans. But if you ask me what the speech was about, I would tell you that it was about the thing that would undergird any effort to address so many of our societal and global challenges: empathy.

That night, he recounted words from our father which I had heard many times in my youth, 'I don't expect the government to solve my problems, but I expect it to understand them.'

We talk a lot these days, and rightly so, about the importance of representation. As the saying goes, you can't be what you can't see. In thinking about the importance of empathy in our lives and our world, I would add a corollary: you can't heal what you don't feel. Empathy is the connective tissue in our humanity. It is the universal language of the soul. The degree to which we can feel determines the degree to which we can relate to one another. And in my experience, the path to empathy is through broadening our understanding of family.

I grew up as Mary Valerie Biden, only sister among Joey, Jimmy and Frankie Biden. My Mom used to say, 'Family is the beginning, the middle and the end. Period.' Our parents taught us that as siblings, we were a gift to one another, and no matter what our disagreements might be, we had to straighten them out at home. Once we ventured outside our front door – we Bidens needed to present a unified front to the world. It was on our little shoulders to make our family proud. And what it took to make our family proud was pretty clear-cut: we were expected to follow what we kids coined 'The Biden Code'. The code was a trio of often-repeated statements, used alternatingly as admonishments or calls-to-action, that clearly delineated reasons why we might be punished, pardoned or praised:

- Take care of each other.
- No one is better than you, but you are no better than anyone else, either. Stand up for what you believe in but do so with civility and respect.
- It's not about how many times you are knocked down, it's about how quickly you get up, because failure in life is inevitable, but giving up is unforgivable.

These tenets fostered in us an appreciation for loyalty, for seeing value in being able to truly understand others, for respectfully resolving conflict, and for developing confidence and resilience in the face of setback or failure. It wasn't until adulthood that we realised that what our parents had chosen to focus their efforts on were, in a sense, way-stations on the road to empathy.

Back then, in the first sign of the political talent that he would display as an adult, my brother Joe instituted what we called 'Family Meetings,' although it was only the four siblings in attendance; our parents never were invited nor did they interfere. Any of us kids could call a meeting for any reason, and when the meeting started, we would get right to the heart of the matter.

'You embarrassed me'. 'You hurt my feelings'. 'You were mean'. These were the typical squabbles of siblings, but we handled them in an atypical way. Our goal was to get the offence out in the open, explain how the transgression made us feel, take responsibility for our actions, stop the hurt the action had caused, mend the rift and move on. We didn't know it at the time, but the empathy we were cultivating within our family could be instructive as we began to operate in a world outside of our family.

For me, those meetings helped build a muscle that I have used over and over again through the years. They helped me realise that empathy isn't just a character trait, it's also a skill that can be learned and improved. I have done my best to give my family, my neighbours and casual acquaintances, and even more fleeting campaign trail encounters the security to just talk, to speak their truth. And as people take that opportunity to talk, I find myself hearing my mother reminding me that 'what goes unsaid is often more important than what is said.' When you really hear both the said and the unsaid, there are many ways to offer comfort: a soft breeze of understanding, a fierce gust of confidence, the relief of a quiet tear.

And it's a skill that our world needs now, possibly more than ever. Only if we are able to understand where others are coming from can we address their concerns in a productive manner and move forward together.

I think one of the reasons that my brother, Joe, has resonated with so many Americans is that he truly shows people how much he cares about them. It is why there was such a feeling of national catharsis when he led our nation in mourning the lives of those lost to COVID-19. He was able to speak personally to the feeling of loss, and, by his words and his example, show that healing – long and hard as the journey may be – will come.

It is why, when he tells a young trans person that 'I see you, and I hear you', those words land so meaningfully; because the world often doesn't.

There is no daylight between the private Joe and the public Joe. He doesn't judge – at least he tries not to – those he doesn't agree with. He not only accepts people for who they are, he also seeks to learn from them. People sense that. And what I sense is that he has taken that gift my parents gave us – clarity about what matters, and the tools for how to listen, love, fight, figure it out and move forward together – and broadened it from our nuclear family to our national family.

The need to see each other as family is so badly needed today. Because if we truly accept one another as family, we make a more empathetic world a reality; one where we see the harm done by lies, the hurt caused by hateful statements, and where we realise there is nothing to be gained by exploitation.

Many years ago, I watched the documentary that many readers may remember: Seven Up (now known as the Up series of documentaries). It has followed the lives of a group of children in England, starting when they were seven years old and checking in on them every seven years thereafter. One of the men featured was asked about the journey of his life and the lives of his fellow participants. He replied with a simple comment that I found absolutely powerful and profound: 'Every life is an incredible act of bravery'. Bravery is more than facing down an enemy; it is also facing up to ourselves. It is the quiet personal courage of just getting up and putting one foot in front of the other, like millions of us do each day. That bravery is no less worthy of celebration than the more public courage we typically celebrate. Every person's struggle is different and deserves respect. When people face life's inevitable challenges, some withdraw, some drink, some want to smash things, and some head to a mosque, temple, or church. We each find our own ways to weep, bleed, despair and camouflage the pain, because most of us do not want to be exposed in our suffering.

Often, we are so preoccupied by our own woes that we fail to appreciate this basic and universal humanity of others. And, lacking curiosity about why someone is acting the way they are, we judge them. We forget to consider that perhaps we are not the only ones who are suffering.

The great leaders are the ones who not only work to heal our suffering, but work to help us recognise the suffering of others. When empathy lies at the heart of our public discourse, politics is more than slogans, speeches, rallies, and television commercials. It is an avenue to decency, respect and the maintenance of the rule of law. It's the way we solve the problems that inevitably arise from living alongside others in a society. It's a way to celebrate the 'act of bravery' that is each of our lives. It's a way to foster greater understanding about how those countless individual acts of bravery not only add up to something much greater, but contribute to something much greater: a community, a society, a world. All of them, in their own way, a family.

Empathy and the Displaced

Niamh Heery

In 2014, I began working on a documentary in relation to displaced populations in Ireland. That year, over sixty million people had been forced to flee their homes. An average of 42,500 people became refugees, asylum seekers, or internally displaced every day.

I searched for people who were experiencing displacement. I found a Syrian refugee, an asylum seeker in Direct Provision, an elderly Traveller woman, an Irish labourer in London and an Offaly turf cutter. While their lives couldn't have been more dissimilar, they each knew the sorrow of the displaced. I sought out these people to hear their stories, but the encounters became more than that.

As a filmmaker, my way of trying to understand intangible statistics is story. Story is universal, present from the moment we're born. Our memories are stories we tell ourselves. It's such a good device through which to explain the world. But for this documentary, I knew I needed to find and show deeper common ground to viewers. So, I delved into the sense memories of the people I met, past facts, figures and politics and straight through their 'third eye,' to the heart of what people were feeling at the time. They spoke so poetically about their inner selves.

A bitterly cold January in the sparsely populated, ageing village of Reyweg in Western Germany. By sundown, the anonymous dwellers of each tidy identical redbrick house had closed their shutters and the roads were empty, save for the sound of Arab music that floated out of one open-windowed home. Yasser, a twenty-one-year-old Syrian refugee had been resettled here with some other young men from war torn Middle Eastern countries. Shisha pipes (traditional Middle Eastern smoking instruments) sat on the sill as our small film crew drank sweet tea before dinner. Yasser floured the kitchen table and the breadmaking began. 'If you ask any Syrian about Syria, the first thing they will tell you about is the bread.' The stateless men fell into a familiar, comfortable rhythm. 'My grandmother makes a fire and sits on the ground. My mother knows how to do it, but now my sisters, they don't know.' Yasser and his friends were kneading and rolling to keep the ancient tradition going, to feel surrounded by family again. The next day as we walked through the village, our cordial greetings were unreturned by curious, uncommunicative locals. Yasser's demeanour was different to the ebullient fraternity I'd seen the previous evening. 'I feel that I am missing something. I don't know if I will keep missing this thing that is maybe home', he lamented, explaining that it wasn't normal to be so cold to your neighbours where he's from, but he is just going to have to adapt. I was struck by the major adjustments he'd already undergone in his young years, and how a small change like returning a 'Hello' on the street was just too much for the community of his new home.

From these experiences I learned that displacement happens when you lose your place in life. You lose part of what you are. Your home, your family, your work, your country. You cling to anything that can bring you back to yourself: a song, a smell, an object. Abstract details of everyday life can trigger the yearning. Bonita, a South African asylum seeker, took me from a damp, cramped Direct Provision bedroom she shared with her mother in inner city Dublin, to Moore Street Market. In my mind, it's the most Dublin of all places but for Bonita the calls of the market women and the smell from the stalls transported her back home. She vividly remembered herself and her (now absent) brother waiting excitedly for her mother to put fruit in a net and squeeze it until sweet juice came out. 'I can almost taste it now,' Bonita whispered with a bittersweet smile.

A Traveller Housing Scheme in North Dublin. Caravans and old wooden wagons sit beside small, spotless cottages. Statues of horses and religious icons adorn pillars. It's tea time for the crew again as Molly and Missy, Traveller women who have been settled here since 1971, explain their method of making tea on the boil of an open fire. They'd simmer it all day and scoop it out by the tin mug for the men when they returned from work. It just doesn't compete with the plastic kettle that sits on the kitchen counter, they tell me. Another simple custom that explains so much of their story. It's February now, still cold. Smoke rises from neighbouring chimneys. 'The house was lovely and comfortable but it was hard to adapt to it. When I see the smoke it brings back everything of the past,' Missy tells me. Soon the two friends are reminiscing about the exact smell of a fire on the side of the road. 'There was a cluster of stars we called the Seven Sisters,' recalls Molly. 'We could be warm in the front of a winter's night and the frost sparkling down on the top of your two shoulders, but you wouldn't feel it because you were brought up that way.' And just like that, a dreamlike, lucid image of home was conjured up. I could see the frost shimmering on a thick woollen shawl, mirroring the stars above. Sitting in the kitchen of a housing estate, I got a real sense of the customs that Molly and Missy had lost.

Match day, London GAA Club, Ruislip. We're greeted by an old Mayo man in a steward's vest who shepherds us towards the parking. We enter the bar past pints of Guinness and photos of sporting legends. Outside the changing rooms, I overhear a coach ordering the team to 'Bate the hell out of them!' The doors burst open and our camera follows Kevin, an emigrant labourer and half-forward for London's senior hurling team, down the tunnel and onto the pitch. *Amhrán na bhFiann* blasts tinnily out from the tannoys. Only afterwards, sitting with Kevin in his impersonal suburban London house share, did I feel like I was in a country other than Ireland at all. Kevin came here, having trained as an estate agent and emerging into the property crisis of 2009. 'We have to move to survive, really. There's nothing really at home for us.' He described roofing houses in the snow, wondering what he was doing with his life. But out on the pitch he felt himself again. The hurl, he said, was 'an extension of my hand since I was three-years-old. The pitch here, it's like being at home when you're out on it.'

For multiple reasons, place is losing permanence and people are in perpetual motion. What people expressed to me, as I accompanied them in their every day and all that lay deep beneath it, gave me a new understanding of how that impermanence affects a person. My last stop on this documentary was a complex contradiction of sorts, but where people were again mourning.

Belmont, Co. Offaly in March. The gorse is beginning to bud. The bogland of Ireland is a fingerprint. It's layered crust a muse for poets, its tradition is the very scent of home for some. I meet Tom and Tommy, two turf farmers who show me their small boglands that provided heat and sustenance to their families for centuries. I can see slices cut through layers, exposing an oversized chocolate cake. But those cuts are the last, made years ago. The rest of the land is overgrown briars. Tom has a wet eye as he describes what the dense brush means to him: more than a loss of fuel, it represents the loss of a way of living.

Perched in front of the sweeping industrial state bog that sits right next door, Tom explains that an EU directive stopped his family from cutting turf for domestic use because of its carbon output. As reddish brown dust settled between the creases of his face, I wanted to know more about what Tom lost. We retired to an old cottage where knotted heather was still used to sweep the floor. A glowing bank of turf enticed me to stop and stare. He fed the fire and the fire got him talking. Tommy sat down and showed me the scythe with a bull's horn handle used by his father, grandfather and himself. His sons would never take hold of it, sighed Tommy. 'They'll have no *grá* for the bog. That era's gone now, it's not in their psyche, in their memory like it's in mine.' They talked more of the community, families helping families sod turf on the bog as long evenings drew in. 'The lark would be rising high in the evening time. They could go up so high you could hardly see them. But that's all part of history now, it's all in the past.' The men heave in the deep earth that burns beside them, fills the floor and is sandwiched between the bricks in the wall of the old cottage. This place feels like the living past. I feel privileged to have experienced it, but it's a living that can't be sustained and because of that, these men and their families have become displaced from their own sense of place while still living there.

Looking back at the film I get that feeling all over again. It's more than nostalgia, it's an instinctual loss felt deep. But it conjures up an urgency now, a realisation that at times of momentous change we all have to lose something. We can't cling to place or we'll all become displaced. Intangible senses and feelings that are hard to verbalise are important to who we are and we should hold them close.

I found poetry in the practice of the people I met. And within that is the transcendent power of empathy. It strips back the layers, the armour of experience and just feels that feeling too, whatever it is. And from that shared space, progress is possible.

Empathy across Generations

Mary Sugrue

One of my abiding memories from my childhood is an image of my grandmother, dressed in an old country apron, standing outside the door of our farmhouse. She was crying as she watched her children, my aunts and uncles, leave after their visit home. Several years later, I witnessed my own mother cry as I pulled away to head back to my adopted home of Boston. Today, leaving is not any easier.

I come from a rural part of County Kerry where emigration has been a part of life for generations. This story is not just mine, but a shared narrative of so many who have said goodbye to the people and places they love.

In my role at the Irish American Partnership, I have heard countless family stories of love and longing, the sorrow of those who left, and the pain of those who remain behind. I have seen the undeniable demonstration of empathy from the descendants of people who once called Ireland home. When they tell their families' stories, you can feel the sorrow of those tearful goodbyes, the heartache as vivid as the day their ancestors left home. The pain of leaving is woven into their family tree, making an indelible mark on each new generation. Our members express empathy not only for their own parents, grandparents, and great-grandparents, but for those who share the same story – the story of longing for a connection. Their empathy propels them forward. It encourages them to understand what their ancestors endured and to take action to honour their roots.

I will tell you here the story of one such man, living in

the flat, wide-open fields that span across the mid-west United States. The view was drastically different from the lush greens and rolling hills of his ancestral home. And while generations removed from Ireland, he always said 'my heart is there', reflecting his deep longing and connection to a place that for many years lived only in his family's stories. He began to visit Ireland regularly. He walks the fields that his family once walked and enjoys long chats with the locals, absorbing all he can about this land that always felt like home. What power to feel that yearning for a place left generations ago and to build a genuine connection after a century apart. I came to understand that his connection to Ireland is not one of nostalgia, it is one of empathy towards the story of his people and the place they once had to leave. Today, he honours that story by supporting the young people who inhabit that place – by trying to give them educational opportunities that his ancestors did not have. His empathy inspires him to pay it forward.

This deep expression of empathy has given me purpose: listening to and appreciating these stories and helping those who tell them make a connection to the places and people they hold dear. I am humbled to know so many people whose empathy inspires a commitment to ensure a bright and inclusive future for Ireland.

In my daily life, I am often reminded of the image of my grandmother crying in her old country apron. Though I did not realise it at the time, that moment was my first understanding of empathy. To me, empathy in practice is helping connect people to the places they call home. It is being there for my fellow emigrant friends as they rush home to say goodbye to a dying family member. It is getting to watch my children enjoy my mother's potato leek soup or eat jelly tots out of my father's hands when I take them home. It is the comfort of chatting with new friends while sipping on a cup of Barry's tea in Boston. Empathy is overcoming the pain of longing and striving for ways in which we can help each other connect.

Today, the story of Ireland includes immigration as well as emigration. With that in mind, we must be intentional with our respect. We must show empathy to those who now call Ireland home, remembering that they too have experienced the pain of leaving behind the people and the places that they love. My grandmother had an old Irish proverb, *Is fusa duine a ghortú na a leigheas* – it is easier to hurt someone than to heal them. We must remember that as we share our homeland with those new to our shores and as we welcome those who return.

Empathy is what propels us forward. It transcends borders and oceans, reminding us that someone from a farther shore might share a similar story. It is what helps us to understand the longing for people and places left behind as well as the grief of those who stay. Empathy is a yearning to make people feel at home.

Our Empathy Story

McDonough Family

Let me preface my writing by stating that I am under no illusion that the McDonough family is more empathetic than any other family as to the understanding of empathy which is best understood in the privacy of one's own heart. However, I am honoured to share my understanding of this critically important human quality.

My three Irish grandparents were born after their families' arrival in the United States in the nineteenth century. My parental great-grandparents came around the middle of the century and my maternal great-grandparents' parents about twenty to thirty years later. My great-grandparents came from Counties Mayo and Sligo, all of strong Catholic backgrounds. My maternal father's side, of English and Dutch decent, came much earlier to the United States in the late sixteenth century. I suspect the impact of the dire circumstances that led all of them to leave their homeland, boldly willing to accept the dangers of crossing an ocean, are traits that might embed empathy in a person. It is also my belief that these qualities, empathy, faith and risk-taking, may have been explicitly or implicitly instilled and passed on to subsequent generations.

Additionally, there were family experiences in Carbondale, Pennsylvania where they settled that further instilled the deep belief that we are here to help one another. Like the risky voyage across the Atlantic Ocean by their parents, my grandparents endured difficult experiences that likely cultivated, perhaps paradoxically, even greater compassion in their hearts.

My maternal grandparents, one Catholic the other Methodist, had their house burned down and their dog shot and killed by the KKK in or around 1924 because they were of a 'mixed' marriage. My other grandfather had the rigorous life of being a coal miner, underpaid and working in hazardous conditions. Instead of hardening their hearts, I believe these life experiences led them to feel more compassion for one another and unique insights.

Of course, this is not always the direction people go when mistreated or experiencing difficult life circumstances. I can only suspect that it was from a willingness to forgive, a deep sense of optimism, and love for one another that helped them persevere through these hardships and actually grow further in character. I can speak with more clarity, a more expansive first-hand account, that these were absolutely the qualities of my parents, no doubt passed down to them from their up-bringing.

Growing up, my brothers, sisters and I were taught to do our best in all endeavours you commit to and help others along the way. However, this help to others, the vulnerable or those left out, was cultivated to come from the heart, while recognising at the same time it is our inherent duty. Importantly, we grew up in a home filled with love and a feeling conveyed from our parents that children were special. I am sure there were countless dinner discussions, day-to-day interactions and not so subtle messaging that provided our parents the opportunity to sow the seeds of empathy in us. As a child of the 1950s and 1960s, the United States was also attempting to impart the notion of service to others as highlighted in John F. Kennedy's Inaugural Address, 'Ask not what your country can do for you, ask what you can do for your country'. These words resonated in our home and in our school, Holy Rosary, in the blue collar community of Claymont, Delaware (also childhood home of President Joe Biden).

My four siblings, my wife, and our children, nieces and nephews all have worked or volunteered in professions that serve others, the community and often the most vulnerable. This includes a sister who was Director of Community Legal Aid of Delaware and, at the same time, volunteered as night manager of a shelter for homeless women; a brother, a former federal prosecutor now represents indigent people; another brother who, having suffered the tragedy of losing a child to cancer after a long battle, started one of the largest childhood cancer philanthropic organisations in the United States, the Andrew McDonough B+ Foundation, for families of children with cancer; another sister, a writer, who has devoted countless hours to helping new immigrants settle in the United States and volunteers with literacy programs; a son who is a decorated Medevac pilot who served nearly eighteen months in Afghanistan risking his own life to save others; a daughter earning a PhD in Urban Affairs and Public Policy while coaching lacrosse at a male juvenile correctional facility; and my wife who turned hairdressing at a nursing home into a quasi-social work position to help comfort these women toward the end of their lives. Both of my sisters adopted a child from a foreign country. Similarly, many of my nieces and nephews also work or volunteer in jobs or initiatives for the betterment of the community.

I worked most of my professional career as a United States Probation Officer and found the most rewarding part of the job was helping returning citizens (many emotionally broken) from prison, reclaim or create for the first time productive, happy lives. The point I would like to highlight is I believe this work described above was strongly driven by a tug on our hearts, a sense of compassion for those in need and oppressed.

My sense of the origins of our empathy can be traced back to our parents, siblings, grandparents, aunts, uncles and cousins. My wife has often commented that 'children are treated special in your family, as gifts'. Although we experienced an appropriately disciplined child-rearing approach, I believe we knew that we were treasured. I believe that to make an adult strong, 'tough' and resilient (and emphatic), a child needs to feel secure growing up, picked up having made a mistake, and able to safely share their fears. This was our experience.

I think another important element of instilling empathy is for a child to grow up in an environment in which families have fun together. Laughter, good-natured Irish mischief, games, relaxing together breeds trust, sacrifice and sharing. 'Fun' helped to tie us together enabling us to see ourselves as part of an essential network of relationships, not isolated individuals. I can recall numerous occasions of great family fun, ranging from beach vacations to sleigh riding, cookouts and simply watching television together. I also have very fond memories of trips to stay with our grandparents and aunts four hours away (the long trips were not so much fun with seven people crammed into a 1965 station wagon). Again, we felt that joy when with our aunts, Marion and Loie, who routinely cleared their schedule to take us and our cousins to Crystal Lake for a day of fun and ice cream (who years later the great-nephews and great-nieces affectionately referred to Loie as 'Duckie'). Or, my grandfather waking me up at 5.00 a.m. as a small child to go fishing on the same lake. Incidentally, my grandparents' house that was burned down was on Crystal Lake and my grandfather, a carpenter, rebuilt it in the exact same spot.

A notable family story relates to my mother's first cousin, Jack Race. Jack now 101-years-old was a pilot in the US Air Force in the Second World War. When in the company of Jack, one is immediately struck by his peaceful nature and non-judgemental spirit. I suspect his superiors in the military recognised the same qualities and selected him to fly the defeated, disgraced German commanders to their surrender. I see him as the ideal conduit for peace. After the war, Jack became an ordained Methodist minister.

Sports were a particularly important formative activity for my brothers and me as well as for my children. The best in youth sports teaches children to sacrifice for their teammate, strive for a common goal, embracing sportsmanship and, of course having fun. Winning and losing both provide an opportunity to connect to another. I am now sixty-six-years-old and I still have vivid memories of these carefree, good times with my family extended family and friends.

All these experiences instilled an empathetic spirit creating a desire to impart it to others, particularly one's children and grandchildren but to perfect strangers too. However, I would not suggest that a 'Norman Rockwell' like childhood is the sole path to empathy. There are plenty of examples one could cite of a people having an epiphany of sorts often after a life-changing experience. I witnessed countless men and women genuinely transform their lives after the trauma of a prosecution and a long prison sentence.

Our family immigrant story continues with the wonderful addition of Yeonjoo, wife of our son, and our two beautiful granddaughters, Lilianna Jia and Isabella Sia. At its core, empathy flows from love.

All Lives Matter

Uchechukwu Helen Ogbu

In writing my contribution, two major quotes by Margaret Mead, an American anthropologist who mainly focused her studies and research on child rearing, personality, and culture resonate with me. The first one is – 'Never doubt that a small group of thoughtful, committed, citizens can change the world. Indeed, it is the only thing that ever has'. *Ionbhá: The Empathy Book for Ireland* is a testament to this quote because the inspiration behind the book is to influence change and bring about a global movement that will inspire the present generation and generations unborn.

Empathy can be defined as the act of understanding, experiencing, and responding to the emotions and thoughts of another person. The two components of empathy are cognitive – understanding another person's feelings or 'putting yourself in someone else's shoes' and emotional – sharing another person's feeling or feeling what other people feel. Empathy is not feeling 'for' but feeling 'with' that person, it is an important element of Emotional Intelligence (EI) which is the act of understanding what others are experiencing as if we are experiencing it ourselves. Empathy is a skill that either comes naturally or is developed, so this movement is timely because it will be a collective effort through the book to encourage those who need to develop the skill, to learn it, practise it, work on it.

This chapter is titled 'All Lives Matter' as an encouragement piece about the power of empathy in our lives for everyone especially the young. I write as a black woman, a migrant and parent of a child born and raised in Ireland. I have experienced empathy; my daughter has experienced it and we know the power that lies with aligning with empathetic people. I have been made to understand that for one to be truly empathetic we need to understand the experience of both worlds. I have experienced life both as a migrant and being 'black Irish' and now understand what it means to be empathetic.

Empathy is a two-way process – you give and take, it should not be one sided. It requires everyone to take turns to connect, listen to and understand one another. It is a shared value of allowing yourself to fully take in another person's emotion to enhance your relationships and allowing yourself to be vulnerable to others to amplify connections. Being empathetic is to feel both the pain of another and know that you are in a position to do something about it.

As a migrant, I want to tell a story of where I come from and where I am going ...

'The Biafran baby – a penny for the Biafra baby'.

Where I am coming from will not determine my destination – it is just another stepping-stone to where I want to get to.

Where I am going is a limitless opportunity, it is a white canvas, but I have to write that story, I have to embrace who I am and write that story myself.

I draw from the values, the beauty, the lessons, the experiences, and I create where it is I want to go to.

But to be able to write and convey my story, my message ... I need a people who are authentic, sincere, empathetic and compassionate.

Thinking about the next fifty years, I may not be around and even if I am around, I will not be active, so what legacy am I leaving behind!

I want to leave behind a legacy of kindness, positivity, connection, courage, vulnerability, compassion and Empathy.

I want to leave behind the core value of Empathy.

The core value that will bridge the divide, change, rebuild and heal our society.

Empathy gives us the ability to see the world through other people's perspectives and feel what they are feeling. It is the basis for the powerful human connection we all long for and brings about a shift that shows the connection, the will to listen, the effort to understand and the push to liaise and work out a solution.

Empathy has shown me that all lives matter!

It means I feel you, recognise and share in your feelings

It means I want to experience putting myself in your shoes – understanding how it feels to be in your place

It means I see your vulnerability but do not consider it as socially unacceptable or weak

It means I will set aside my own ways and not only 'love and care for self' but also care for others

It means I understand that everybody's pain, fear, story is very real to them

It means I believe your story and will not sweep your emotions to one side

It means I will not make remarks such as 'stop complaining' and 'be grateful' for being 'here' thereby deepening the sense of disconnection you already feel

It means I feel you; I hear you and will work with you to come up with a solution and the way forward for the general good of our society.

Empathy Matters because:

It makes 'all lives matter'

It makes us observant, curious and ask questions to be well informed

It helps us communicate and makes us listen more to others and expand our opinion

It helps us realise that we need each other and to look out for one another

It helps us recognise our own feelings – a prerequisite for empathising with others

It helps us understand others and take an active interest in their issues

It makes us imagine ourselves in another's shoes

It helps us discover a shared commonality, even if we hold different beliefs

It helps us challenge racism, prejudice, binds commonalities and expand our moral universe

It helps us become a people who believe in faith, kindness, love, care for our neighbours and understand that not even one of us is an island to itself

It helps us realise that every one of us holds a piece of what is required to build the world we can all survive and co-exist

It helps us develop, build and practise emotional intelligence skills

It prevents us from labelling people as the other, problems, enemy-drawing lines that prevent us from growing as a unified society

It helps us talk together, build bridges and move the country forward

It helps us leverage diversity by embracing the different cultures and recognising that we all bring different talents, skills, and opportunities

It makes us treat everyone with respect, listen, understand and interact with them in ways that match their needs and feelings

It makes us act on needs and become problem-solvers,

showing compassion by relieving others' suffering and changing their situations

It allows people to build social connections with others. By understanding what people are thinking and feeling, people can respond appropriately in social situations

It helps create an empowering environment where everyone feels welcome and thrives to achieve their goals

It helps us incorporate and develop the three Hs dimensions of learning – hearts, hands, and head

It helps us experience other people's darkness and collaborate with them to turn on the right light which will illuminate their situations

It helps us meet people, understand the barriers they face and break down those barriers

It helps you learn to regulate your own emotions and be non-judgemental

It promotes high self-esteem, strong sense of self and reduces our loneliness

Empathy establishes our role as human beings and is the key that can unlock the door to our kindness and compassion

It fosters trust, builds relationships, breaks down barriers, shatters stereotypes and bridges the lines of cultural divides

It helps promote and achieve integration, inter-culturalism and diversity

It helps us create an equitable, resilient, and united society.

Reflect

In every neighbourhood there is a mixture of white, brown, black and mixed-race people but have you taken time to engage with your neighbour to know what makes them different? Are they really different? Or are we engulfed in our stereotyping tendencies? What would you say? What will you do? What action are you willing to take today?

Would you consider yourself to be empathetic?

On an average day, how often do you listen, understand and support someone to overcome challenges or issues?

What do we need to change?

I challenge us to convert the lack of empathy in the society to solutions, ideas, pathways, initiatives and create vessels of empathy.

I close my chapter with one of Mead's quotes which says that male and female personality characteristics are not necessarily determined by heredity, but by society and cultural conditioning. She says – 'Children must be taught how to think, not what to think'. *Ionbhá: The Empathy Book for Ireland* is all about teaching the youth about empathy and its power in shaping the world into a welcoming and compassionate place where we can all co-exist. I believe that beliefs are picked up as children and from the society, so we need to teach the young and make a conscious effort to inculcate empathy in their belief and value systems, so that it becomes a habit. It is just like going to the gym, we need to train ourselves, practise, bring in a little every day and keep doing that activity to make it easier, fluid and a habit which then becomes our default.

Let us engage in unconditional positive regard – it means that our regard for ourselves and for others should always be positive, even in the absence of 'conditions'. People do not have to do anything to receive empathy or compassion from you, all we need is to accept and love one another as we love ourselves, extending compassion and grace without conditions.

People are like plants, they need soil, water and sun to blossom. Some are oaks, pines, willows, and some are bamboo ... We all have different ways of doing things and need to understand our differences. We grow differently and need different types of nurturing to sprout. Some of us need understanding, compassion and acceptance for us to blossom and bloom.

We need Empaths who are not just there to show pity but people who understand, who have those characteristics of respect, value, loving, giving. We want a generation of people in Ireland who are united, have emotional intelligence and are compassionate ... we want to leave a legacy that will stand the test of time, that will impact everyone.

We need to teach empathy from the cradle and nurture the children who become youths and future leaders of tomorrow on how to work as a team, play together, support each other, solve problems together without any bias but look beyond colour, religion, creed or orientation. Together, through this book and movement, we can make the world what we want it to be and build a better future for our children. I stand with all the contributors – keep believing! For others, are you ready to take that step? It is not easy but if you open yourself up, you will receive, and we will transform this vision board of empathetic Ireland to reality.

There are key moments in one's life that shape the core of who you are, who you become … Empathy informs those key moments and leads to freedom, it creates compassion which makes all lives matter.

Can We Teach History Without Historical Empathy?

Sarah-Anne Buckley

Historical empathy has, since the 1980s, been a controversial topic for historians. It has raised questions around bias and objectivity, the idea that we 'need' to be distant from the sources we use and investigate. How can we interview someone who spent most of their life in an institution without empathising? How can we research the topic of rape or domestic violence without understanding the power and vulnerability it exposes? Even when we look at the state, how can we understand it without understanding the people who held positions of power, the people who legislated? And it is our role as historians, as students of history, to make connections, bring new insights and push to understand society in the past to improve society today.

While we may not always call it Historical empathy, with the emergence of social history, the history of emotions, transnational history and gender history (to name but a few), we are more interested than ever in how an experience or event felt, not only the narrative or details of what occurred.

I would argue that contextualising how someone felt in a particular time or place, being aware of our own position and personal connection, and searching for and advocating for an individual or group that has previously been ignored is a critical part of connecting with our past. It is also a crucial part of understanding our present.

I wasn't always conscious of why I was studying a certain

topic or using a particular method to do so, but, looking back, everything I have researched has been deeply personal. I remember the first time I took a course on 'Radical Politics in Twentieth Century Ireland' as an undergraduate and realised the ideas and ideals of first wave feminists were still the ideas and ideals, second and third wave feminists were seeking to answer and explore. I realise now that I always chose areas that were underdeveloped, that were the 'tip of the iceberg'. Whether social history, feminist history, oral history – the importance of empathy and care could not be under-estimated.

I have seen the impact the growth of gender history, transnational history and the history of emotions has had on students – and I have felt more connected with each personal story or connections these approaches bring. I have watched activists push the boundaries of scholarship and research, and students push their lecturers, and it can only bring more colour and life to our work. It is my job to make them contextualise – it is their job to challenge me, and they certainly do.

Sometimes the documents and primary sources we are addressing can be traumatic – not only listening to someone speak of their individual experience but reading a court document or a press report. Often, it is the lack of empathy in these documents that causes the most distress. Or what has been erased or omitted.

The great white men of history still hold a strong position, but the women, the brown and the black people, the children, the poor, the queer and the often marginalised are pushing through – in their testimonies, their songs, building their own archives. My students care about how it felt, they want to understand the positionality of individuals. Whether that is a person with power, or someone who is vulnerable to that power. Every factor that affects our life course today – our gender, where we grew up, how we grew up, our education and experiences (both positive and negative), our sexuality, our hobbies – these factors affected the lives of those who lived in the nineteenth century, or before – whether the language used was the same or not. When we realise this, when we look empathetically, and rigorlessly, we reveal how beautifully complex the ordinary and the extraordinary moments were.

Can we teach history without historical empathy?

We can, but I don't think we should.

Northern Dilemmas

Alan and Elaine Smith

1974

What do you think our friends would think
if I went out with you?
I'm not too sure, but it feels right,
let's try it for a while.

How do you think our parents will feel
if we get married too?
They'll not be sure if we'll be safe,
they'll worry what we'll do.

What do you think the priest will do
if we walk down the aisle?
He'll grit his teeth and wish us well
behind a holy smile.

2022

You know I hate those stereotypes
that Northern Ireland has.
'Love across the barricades',
and all that sentimental jazz.

You know I hate being pigeon-holed,
constricted by our past.
We fell in love,
that was enough.

Your past is gone, and mine is too.
We're still the same somehow,
but our children are the future,
they have no labels now.

What will we do if we have kids?
What do you think they'll be?
We'll just be sure to love them well
and teach them to be free.

Free from fear and violence
is what we hope for them.
It matters less what we believe,
we believe in them.

A Wing-Back and a Prayer

A Protestant Player's Journey through the GAA

Colin Regan

My father placed at the bottom of our lane the shell of an old Hiace van to provide shelter for my two brothers and I as we waited for the bus to ferry us to school.

There was nothing unusual in this. My father found use in many things that others had discarded. What was unusual was that each morning we watched and waved as the bus carrying our friends and neighbours passed by en route to the local national school in Tullaghan on Leitrim's coastline. We instead travelled to Ballyshannon in Co. Donegal to obtain a faith-based education that reflected our Protestant upbringing.

It wasn't far geographically. Just 15km. But psychically, it was a significant journey. It marked us out as different. This has the potential to dislocate a youngster whose understanding of the world is framed by one's identity and relationship with one's peers. However, if such differences are understood and accepted then they have the potential to foster an appreciation that diversity is part of the tapestry of life. Thankfully, our family celebrated the similarities we shared with our neighbours as much as our only real difference: our denomination.

While my primary and secondary education took me to another county and province, my local GAA club, Melvin Gaels, helped to root me in my community. It exposed me to a deeper understanding of our community's Family Tree. Such knowledge in rural Ireland was in part accessed through shared schooling and worship. My awareness of family connections – both between people and their geographical or social footprint – was helped by my father's work as a silage, hay and turf contractor. This meant that my siblings and I worked the land and sat at the dinner tables of households far beyond the immediate surroundings of our small farm. But my involvement in the Melvin Gaels club further layered my appreciation of our place and its people. I played with brothers, cousins, uncles, as their parents, grandparents, aunts, neighbours, watched from the sidelines or helped to run the club. It broadened my world and enriched it through shared experiences.

One example resonates deeply. It was 1987, I was eleven and Galway was hosting the U14 *Féile na nGeal* festival. Myself and my team-mate Aidan Dolan were housed by a wonderful family from the Cortoon Shamrocks club where we played in the fields with their scatter of children until we ran out of daylight. It has become one of those sun-kissed memories by which I define my youth. On the Sunday morning, a mass was being held in the cathedral in Galway, the largest building I had ever seen. All participating clubs were queuing outside in their finery, waiting to be called to their respective pews. I was excited and apprehensive – I had never been to mass before (bar attending some funerals with my father) and didn't want to do the wrong thing.

I'm not sure what triggered our mentors, Jimmy Phelan and Patsy McGovern, but they looked at me and then each other, and said: 'Jesus, what about young Regan?' They asked if I would like to attend the service and offered to find a Protestant church instead. I wanted to stay with my friends naturally and explained that I was looking forward to the ceremony but didn't really know what to do. My friends reassured me they would keep me right and, to much mirth and a little myrrh, we rehearsed receiving communion in our pew before our turn came around. It all seems so simple now, but there is a reason I can access this memory in technicolour: it meant a lot to me. I was one of the tribe and they had my back.

The flip side of this was the rare occasions I experienced alienation in the GAA due to my religion. The first time was during one of my first seasons playing with our club's adult team (at an age that our rules now, rightly, deem too young for a teenager to go up against grown men). I had the engine of a Massey Ferguson 135 and was giving one of those grown men a torrid time. Having landed a point, I was returning to my position when he looked at me and said: 'you're nothing but an Orange Bastard Regan'. I was familiar with the term. It was thrown about regularly while in secondary school in Raphoe in Donegal where our uniform identified us as pupils of the largely Protestant Royal & Prior school. While walking the streets of the town it was thrown like a stone by the occasional group of lads from the local vocational school. It was hurled from sidelines and on the field when we played in the Donegal schools soccer league. Especially when we won.

I had also twice heard it spat at my father in pubs in our locale. I was very young the first time, maybe ten. It was Christmas and our family had gathered in The Diamond Bar in Tullaghan to welcome home my older brothers who were working the sites in London and Germany in the 1980s. I don't know how the offending party – a group of northern men drinking at the bar – learned of Dad's religious leaning and I never asked. I just remember the words cutting like a knife through the jovial sounds of the festive season before all hell broke loose.

After the game against our neighbouring club, my opponent had the decency to seek me out and apologise. He said he had spoken out of frustration and hoped I did not take it personally. I didn't. I could see that his apology was genuine. His words came from a place of ignorance rather than hate. I ended up playing long enough to have regrets over things I too have said and done in the heat of a game.

Nonetheless, I enjoy being a minority in the GAA. The Protestant. Being outed as such still has the capacity to surprise, which makes me smile. In the late Noughties as part of his eponymous summer school, I chaired a discussion in Aughawillan's Community Centre on the author John McGahern's depiction of the GAA. One of the contributors spoke about 'The Big House' trope in Irish literature and the unfamiliarity of Irish Protestantism with the GAA. Outing myself, I warned against the dangers of stereotypes, and pointed out that a member of Leitrim's famous Connacht winning team of 1994, George Dugdale, also kicked with his left foot. Afterwards, an old farmer who could have stepped out of the pages of one of McGahern's short stories approached me and quietly noted that he found it remarkable that 'our people' could end up playing with the GAA. He said to keep it up.

I feel privileged to have represented my club and county. The GAA community have opened their homes and hearts to me and have made available opportunities that have defined and enriched my life. Providence has allowed me to pursue a career with the association, and perhaps it's no coincidence that diversity and inclusion falls within my remit as GAA Community & Health manager.

When the GAA in 2019 launched our new manifesto 'Where We All Belong' I considered it a call to action more than a state of play. The perspective and contribution of minority groups will enrich what is one of the finest amateur sporting associations in the world and a priceless contributor to Irish life. The experience of the pandemic bore this out. We are a games-based organisation but when our games stopped, our people didn't. They rallied around those most impacted in our communities and by the height of the first lockdown in May 2020, almost 20,000 GAA volunteers were distributing essential goods, groceries and medications, to nearly 35,000 people forced to self-isolate due to Covid-19. That is empathy in action.

Gaelic Games are our shop-window and they are wonderful things. They elevate us above the mundane of everyday life. When they were taken from us, we were shocked by the degree to which we missed the pageantry, the mastery, the rivalry and the coming together of our tribe to celebrate our culture. But the GAA's greatest assets are our people, and we should never forget that no matter their creed, their colour, their orientation, their disability, their nationality, their club or county.

Closer to Home

Eoin, Róisín & Brendan Dolan

Dad has always been a kind and generous person. He has given so much to those closest to him. But looking back through the years, this extended far beyond his inner circle of friends and family, to strangers, to people living far away from us across the world.

It started from an early age, sitting around watching TV at home with my brother Brendan and our little sister Róisín. Dad would watch the end of 'The Den' (Ireland's main kids TV show) with us most days when he got home from work. His favourite character was Dustin the Turkey. We think it was because Dustin was a bit of a chancer, and he was from Dublin, the same as Dad. At six o'clock it was always time for the news. Famine, war, social unrest, sadly recurring, almost constant daily stories. While some people would stick with a particular narrative, Dad always tried to dig deeper into a story and find what lay at its core.

After the September 11 atrocities in 2001, violence and revenge were in everyone's thoughts particularly in Ireland, where there are such strong ties to the United States. Like most people in our country, Dad was horrified by the attacks and wanted to see justice for the victims and their families. However, he could also look at things from a different angle.

Almost overnight, it felt Afghanistan became the target for people's rage. A country thousands of miles away ruled by the brutal Taliban regime, another stage set for war. Bombs would be dropped on people's homes, many people would die but in the red mist that descended after 9/11, in most people's minds there seemed to be no other option.

Mam and Dad to this day are committed pacifists. As children, they took us on peace marches at the height of the Troubles. In their eyes, this conflict was no different. How was killing more innocent people going to change anything? Whether it's with a precision guided missile or a car bomb, the result is the same. Their empathy lay with families, just like ours, in a foreign country who would soon have their lives turned upside down as a result of this conflict. Brendan and I went with Dad up to Dublin for a hastily organised peace march to show solidarity with the people of Afghanistan, as well as for the victims of the September 11 attacks. At Parnell Square, we met our aunties Monica and Theresa, two of Dad's sisters (he is the youngest of ten by the way!). They have always been role models in our family for developing empathy skills and advocating for social justice. Michael D. Higgins gave an impassioned speech for Ireland to remain neutral and not to support the war effort as other European countries were now doing.

After the speakers were finished, we slowly made our way down through Dublin's city centre. There was a small crowd of us, difficult to tell from memory but certainly no more than a few hundred. What stood out to me the most from that day was the reaction of certain individuals observing the march as we passed by. The remarks ranged from casual expletives to shouts of support for America. On the car journey home I had plenty of questions for Dad. He was thoughtful in his response: 'Put yourself in their shoes. They're angry and frightened. We have to understand where they're coming from if we're to have any hope of making them see our side of the argument'. One of our father's greatest strengths is his ability to break down complex world issues into the individual interactions of day-to-day life.

Having empathy for others, particularly those that don't agree with you, is the key to making this work.

Dad has a unique ability to make a connection with people of every age and social background. He has a learned understanding that we all strive for the same things in life; love, security and somewhere to belong. This is demonstrated in an immeasurable number of modest, uncomplicated everyday acts, from giving something to someone in need to simply trying to make you smile. For kids it was usually the yes-no game or a magic trick he always does, the one where he makes a coin disappear and then reappear behind your ear. For older people it was almost always one or two of his terrible jokes!

Brendan, Róisín and my greatest tribute to both our parents will be to have empathy and compassion in our hearts for our family, friends and community in our day-to-day lives. To the people we find common ground with and those we disagree with, may love and positivity endure.

Who Am I to Judge?

Fr Peter McVerry

I once got a letter from a seven-year-old boy, with €50 in it. He wrote that he had just made his first holy communion and wanted to share what he had collected with children who were less fortunate than himself. He got a very special letter of thanks.

Five years later, I got another letter from the same boy, this time with €100 in it (inflation!). He had just made his confirmation. He got another special letter of thanks! I thought: here is a boy growing up in very different circumstances to those of most of the young people I work with.

I gave a birthday card to a young homeless boy, who was living in one of our hostels. He started crying.

'Why are you crying?' I asked.

'I've never had a birthday card before,' he said.

One young man grew up to be a very professional shop-lifter. He told me of how, when he was seven or eight, his parents would regularly keep him out of school to go shop-lifting with them. His role was to create a tantrum to distract the security guards while his parents would take what they wanted off the shelves. Shoplifting became a normal part of his life. He is now in jail.

Another young man was a persistent thief. Nothing was safe when he was around. But he told me of how his alcoholic parents spent all their evenings (and their money) in the pub. There was rarely any food in the house. The ESB bill wasn't paid so their home was in darkness after the sun went down.

They would often come home late at night, drunk, and have an almighty row, shouting and screaming at each other, which might go on until 2 a.m. or 3 a.m. At nine years of age, he decided he would leave his home every day when it got dark, and stay out all night to avoid the fighting. He had to fend for himself, and to get food and clothes, he had to take whatever opportunities came across his path. He is now receiving counselling in rehabilitation.

Another young man told me that, when he was twelve, his alcoholic parents would send him out each night into prostitution and he had to bring back money or get a beating. He started taking drugs to blot out the memories. Over the years, he built up a drug debt which he could not pay. He was shot dead.

We all have the same dreams, the same hopes, the same desires but each person's life experience, their story, is different. I imagine two babies, born at the same time in the same maternity hospital, lying side by side in their cots. One will grow up to be a judge, the other will grow up to be an armed robber. Their future is not determined by their DNA! No, their future is largely shaped by their experiences growing up. We tend to judge people by their behaviour, or by what they say. But there is always a reason behind their behaviour or their attitudes. I have known many people who have caused a lot of trouble and hurt to others. But I have never known a person who has caused trouble to others who wasn't already troubled themselves. I have never known a person who caused hurt to others who wasn't already hurting inside themselves. Empathy means trying to put myself in someone else's shoes, to try to understand how and why another thinks, feels and behaves as they do. When we understand that, we see people differently. We can still judge their behaviour, of course, but we will stop judging the person.

Our lives are like pieces of a beautiful tapestry, but we can only recognise the beauty of the tapestry when we put all the pieces together. Each person is a story, a beautiful story, but sometimes a very sad story, and we are all enriched by hearing their story. When we listen attentively to another person's story, our shared vulnerabilities unite us and we form a bond which changes or strengthens our relationship to them. We look at them differently, we gaze on them in wonder.

I have listened to the stories of many homeless people. We can often mistakenly believe that most homeless people's live are not very interesting or worth listening to. But many homeless people want to tell their story because they know that their story is uniquely personal and worth telling. In fact, I find homeless people's stories exceptionally interesting and often fascinating. Some of their stories bring tears to my eyes and I often wonder could I have survived what they have experienced. As they try, again and again, to affirm their own dignity as persons, in the face of so many forces telling them that they are of little value, homeless people are the real defenders of human rights.

Yesterday's Enemies

Saoirse Egan

Who knew the world's head would be turned by a carol? Who could have thought that one frozen evening lanterns would be lit in the trenches as soldiers began to sing songs of their homeland, that celebrating the holiday would capture the attention of their rivals, and of the world? Many will know this story, the Christmas Truce, more intimately than I ever will, but my journey through this story is one I would like to share, as it has caused me to explore the concept of empathy in a way I hadn't previously.

Over a hundred years after this event, the Great War seems very distant, and this story more like a legend or fable than real life, but it did happen and it was real and it changed the lives of thousands that day. Remembering this, the story becomes much more than just heart-warming, it swells into the grand compelling story it was, that took place in one of the worst hours of our history and reaches us this far into the future.

This story is, without a doubt, one of the most phenomenal of its age; I think there is great beauty in the coming together of the soldiers, despite everything that would keep them apart, that in spite of their awful conditions and exhausted minds, they were able to recognise the other in themselves, and rejoice in a new day together.

This story's beginning seems so simple, and yet its result was to such a scale that it still inspires awe today with the distance of over a century, due to the empathy the soldiers demonstrated.

Once empathy arises, peace becomes a possibility, as empathy is the root of peace, and empathy can be much easier to find in ourselves than peace when things feel out of control. This is what is so special about this story; the soldiers, in the midst of war, found something in common between them and were happy to end the fighting there. All the animosity and fear evaporated, in nearly no time at all.

How though? Well, when war broke out in late July 1914, the recruits never expected it to last through the coming Christmas. However, as the months closed in and winter arrived, it became clear that the warfare would extend well past the new year. When requests for an official Christmas truce were refused, the soldiers had to continue the daily battle, suffering at the will of their superiors.

After weeks of miserable, soaking weather down in the trenches, the soldiers were ready to drop, aching for home, for any respite or chance to stand down. Many were not much older than sixteen, and there wasn't enough weaponry to go around, leaving many defenceless. They were terrifying, harrowing months and Christmas that year had a hungry feeling to it, but as the rain froze, cloaking the beaten ground in fresh white dustings of frost, the cold air became subtly woven with the sounds of German singing. *Stille Nacht. Heilige Nacht.*

What wonder, and confusion, the armies must have felt, what surreality they were faced with as the song began to grow with the joining voices. Graham Williams of the Fifth London Rifle Brigade, described it for us; 'First the Germans would sing one of their carols and then we would sing one of ours, until when we started up "O Come, All Ye Faithful" the Germans immediately joined in singing the same hymn to the Latin words *Adeste Fideles.* And I thought, well, this is really a most extraordinary thing – two nations both singing the same carol in the middle of a war.'

After long months, despite the order to continue fighting, the worst war in their history came to a standstill, and the harsh noises of the fight faded into the background as they focused in on the treasured melody. While surrounded by the shell-shocked earth and the frail hopes of their fellow soldiers, these men had had the courage to raise their voices and sing. In many areas along the Western Front, the trenches could be as close as 50–300 yards away, a hair-raising proximity in a war zone, but one that allowed the soldiers on this evening to form a truce as they shouted Christmas wishes across the wasteland separating them.

There was magic in this moment, something very special about how both armies stopped and listened, and something shifted as the connection grew. Private Frederick Heath wrote home of a 'night [that] wore on to dawn – a night made easier by songs from the German trenches, the piping of piccolos, and from our broad lines laughter and Christmas carols.' Both sides gradually joined the festivities and empathy and fellow-feeling was fostered between the Allied Forces and the German men.

The next morning, the anticipation was palpable among the soldiers, unsure whether or not the truce could be held. Ducking in and out of the trenches, they gauged their opponents' sincerity, until they felt safe to emerge. Soon the ground was milling with hundreds of soldiers, fixing their trenches, gathering friends, comrades who had died on the field, and reaching out to their counterparts.

Many Germans spoke English, some had even been employed in London when the war broke out, and soon souvenirs, photos of home, were being brought out as the soldiers began to share their stories with each other. They exchanged food and cigarettes, and gave each other tokens of buttons and hats to remember the morning by.

Footballs, and some repurposed ration tins, were brought out and goals were made of hats, coats, bags, anything they could use. The ground was frozen, uneven and wasted, but the soldiers threw themselves enthusiastically into the game. Teams came together, and in the frosty morning air, No Man's land rang with the sounds of shouting and cheering, pounding footsteps and victorious laughter. Cameras, intended to take pictures of gory victories, captured the moment, men and boys, enemy soldiers, side by side, playing football and sharing their stories. Their coats were different, but it didn't seem to matter; they were the same.

Lieutenant Johannes Niemann remembered the football game for an interview in the 1960s, the men 'keeping rigorously to the rules, despite the fact that it only lasted an hour and that we had no referee. A great many of the passes went wide, but all the amateur footballers, although they must have been very tired, played with huge enthusiasm. Us Germans really roared when a gust of wind revealed that the Scots wore no drawers under their kilts – and hooted and whistled every time they caught an impudent glimpse of one posterior belonging to one of "yesterday's enemies". But after an hour's play, when our Commanding Officer heard about it, he sent an order that we must put a stop to it. A little later we drifted back to our trenches and the fraternisation ended.'

These unprecedented events took place in many forms over almost two-thirds of the Western Front that Christmas, not in one site alone. The truce was not universal but an estimated 100,000 Irish, British, French, German and Scots men took part in this series of unofficial truces that lasted anywhere from hours to days in different parts of the Front.

Their superiors were furious, concerned that this would damage 'fighting morale', forcing the men to end the truce and return to their trenches, and taking great measures to prevent a sequel. This strong and unwelcome show of authority was well out of step with the troops' feelings, and cost their superiors much respect. It was with scowls and curses that many of them returned to their miserable trenches, to fight a war they no longer believed in, against soldiers they now saw as men such as themselves.

While the war was punctuated with other short truces, none neared this one in terms of length or effect, making the Christmas truce as unique as it is extraordinary. I really find it to be like something one might find in a fictional world, having peace and humanity break through the clutches of such strong antagonistic influences. In seeking the comfort of a Christmas carol, the soldiers brought into being the comfort of home, and this resonated with their enemy, who went on to find brothers and friends. They had allowed themselves to see the other for what they were: determined young men, doing their best in a war for their country.

This story has spread through and beyond a war, and reached us, over a century into the future. Empathy does matter, it does make a difference. In the vast expanse of the First World War, empathy brought a hundred thousand soldiers, mortal enemies, together. If there is anything we can take from the war, it's that we can't ever have another like it, and if there is something we can take from this story it is the unbelievable reach of empathy into our hearts, and what we are capable of in that collective mindset. Empathy wasn't originally something that had to be learned; it is a fundamental instinct that allowed us to survive when survival depended on relating with others in our group. We are interdependent independents; our lived experience is enhanced by knowing how to live among others. Surely it does not require the depths of a war to have our hearts open like this?

This stunning story represents in a way few others can, how reaching out is not a weakness, nor a retreat, but sometimes a radical act of courage. Empathy is a powerful instrument for peace and unity, so much so that after just a few hours, a veteran could remember the opposing army as 'yesterday's enemies', as people who thought to bring a football to a war.

The True Power of Sport to Really Connect

Hugo MacNeill

Sport has been a very big part of my life. Playing rugby for Ireland at a time when we were winning international championships was special. We also won a few wooden spoons (when you were beaten by all the other countries).Travelling around the country gave you a great connection to people. Hearing them tell you where they were on one of those championship days was magical. You knew you were at the heart of something big and your own experience was added to by all the wonderful stories of other peoples' match days. When you are playing you are somewhat insulated from this until the match itself and the aftermath. In addition to the successful times there were the hard times when you had the opposite emotions. Being whitewashed by the All Blacks on the 1983 British and Irish Lions tour was tough. Being hammered 33–6 at Twickenham in 1988. When the English crowd were so amazed at what was happening they were moved to song. The only song they all knew was 'Swing Low Sweet Chariot'. As we stood under the posts awaiting the conversion of another English try the song echoed around the great Twickenham Stadium. It has haunted me ever since. Only joking. Or only partially joking.

But the great thing about sport is that it is sometimes much bigger than sport. Two particular experiences stand out. The first was centred around the Irish Rugby tour to South Africa in 1981 (when the apartheid regime was very much in power) and the second was the Peace International in 1996, post the IRA bombing of London's Canary wharf.

I made my international debut in 1991. I had dreamed, like many others, of actually playing rugby for Ireland and now it was a dream come true. At the end of the season, there was a tour to South Africa. It was highly contentious whether the Irish team should go and it literally split the country and the rugby community. In the same way that some years later the Roy Keane episode in Saipan provoked a similar split. We were all asked would we travel and confirm our availability or not. In fairness to the Irish Rugby Football Union there was absolutely no pressure put on any player to go. It was our own decision and whatever the outcome it would be respected. I read a lot about it. I was a student in Trinity at the time where there was a very active Anti-Apartheid grouping affiliated to the national organisation under the leadership of Kadar Asmal who was a law professor and was to go on to become a Minister in President Nelson Mandela's government. I read a lot of what they wrote. On the other hand there was a very loud public element advocating 'keeping politics out of sport'. The more I read and the more people I spoke to, I came to the conclusion that in South Africa politics was very much entwined in sport. Few if any black or coloured players selected, segregation in the stadiums and so on ... I got lots of letters and calls urging me to do one thing or the other. I had set up a campus branch of the third world charity GOAL in Trinity College and there was a strong connection to black Africa. But what really swung my decision was the black and coloured leaders in South Africa asking us not to come. The Afrikaners might not have liked being economically curtailed in international trade. But, they really hated not being able to see their beloved Springboks play in Pretoria, Johannesburg and all the other great cities of South

Africa. Therefore I along with three other players – Tony Ward, Donal Spring, Moss Keane – decided not to go.

I have never regretted the decision and, if anything, that conviction grew stronger. I had the privilege of spending a couple of years at Oxford University. There were a number of South Africans in the rugby team and they were pretty liberal in their outlook. I will never forget saying goodbye to one of them, Chris Hugo Hammond, a giant of a man who was a doctor who went on to work in the most deprived areas in South Africa. 'Do come and see us' were his parting words 'but not on a rugby tour!' If you had told me then that fourteen years later a black President Mandela was going to present the World Cup to a South African captain I would not have believed it. He had shocked the Springbok team before the final by appearing in their dressing room dressed in a Springbok cap and jersey. Long-time symbols to the black and coloured communities of Apartheid South Africa. Fast forward to 2019 and you have a black South African captain receiving the rugby World Cup. Amazing from the perspective of that earlier time. But not thankfully viewed from the perspective of today.

The Peace International of 1996 was to have a very strong line of connection to the events in South Africa. I had played eight years for the Irish team across a period of extreme turbulence and suffering in Northern Ireland. When I started playing rugby for Ireland one frequently heard that it was great that players from all over the island played together without the troubles ever being mentioned. I found that a bit strange. If you have a teammate whom you completely trust and respect in the cauldron of international rugby, then surely you can have respectful conversations to really get a sense of what they thought. If not how do you expect people coming out of polarised and divided neighbourhoods to do so. So we did talk. Principally with my great friend Trevor Ringland, but others from Northern Ireland as well. I learned so much about the perspectives of unionism. The great thing about the rugby is that it brings people together from all parts of this island without threatening anyone's sense of identity. Celebrating difference in that an Irish team is inconceivable without the Ulster component (many of them situated in Northern Ireland). BT Sport made a documentary on how rugby brought people together on this island, independent of their political or constitutional allegiances. Two recent captains, former close teammates, and British & Irish Lions Brian O'Driscoll from Dublin and Rory Best (CBE) from Ulster were talking and Brian expressed his confusion. 'Rory you play for Ireland and yet are British at the same time'.

'That's right,' replied Rory.

'I just don't get that', said Brian without in any way seeking to be provocative or rude. I would respectfully say this attitude reflects that of many in the Republic who have real difficulty understanding the concept of genuinely being British and Irish at the same time. It echoes the well-known point emphasised by Ulster poet John Hewitt when expressing the various components of his identity 'I always maintained that our loyalties had an order to Ulster, to Ireland, to the British archipelago, to Europe and that anyone who skipped a step or missed a link falsified the total'.

When the IRA bombed Canary Wharf I called Trevor Ringland. I suggested a Peace International where we brought the best players in the world to Dublin to play Ireland and inviting all Irish supporters who wanted peace to come and back it. It was a year after the extraordinary events of South Africa winning the world cup and the images of President Mandela (wearing his Springbok cap and jersey) and Springbok captain,

Francois Pienaar, went around the world. I knew that we had to get one of the leading Springboks – ideally Francois – to come and captain the visiting Barbarians team. We had six weeks to organise it. The response was extraordinary. Word came from Francois that he was in and did not want a penny. That was organised by John Robbie the former Irish scrum half who had gone on the 1981 tour. He had stayed in South Africa with his family afterwards and hosted a radio show that was a very outspoken critic of the Apartheid regime – attracting a number of death threats to those who would have liked him silenced. Many of the best players in the world came to Dublin. The band the Corrs (who came from Dundalk on the border) asked could they come and play. They interrupted a European tour to fly in, set up band on the North Terrace and then fly out. Many people came who had never been to a rugby match.

There were no flags or anthems. The guests of honour were children who had lost parents and siblings to the violence. Darren Baird who lost both his parents and sister in the IRA bombing of a fish and chip shop on the Shankill Road, Tommy Mullen, whose brother was killed in a reprisal attack at Greysteel a week later and Gareth Bouldsworth (whose best friend Tim Parry was killed in the IRA bombing of Warrington.) The minute's silence with these young people was so powerful. They were so young and so small especially as they were introduced to the visiting players. No one should have to go through what they went through, but particularly as children. At the end of the game, where the result was incidental, the visiting Barbarians team who included some of the great names of world rugby, Phillippe Sella, David Campese, Rory Underwood and so on, did a lap of honour. The crowd rose to their feet and gave them a long-standing ovation to thank them for lending their names to those who were working for peace on this island. I was lucky enough to have had many great days in that Lansdowne Road stadium but nothing could ever match the emotions I felt as I watched this lap of honour. An extraordinary event, pulled together in just six weeks and driven forward by an overpowering sense that it was the right thing to do. As Trevor always says, 'you can push the right buttons or the wrong ones with people and get dramatically different outcomes'. Let's just keep pushing as many right ones as we can.

Best Way to Human

Imelda May

Empathy's catching
haven't you heard!?
practice it often
you'll be riddled with caring
for lobsters and crabs
classed sentient beings
brought to our senses
by crustaceans screaming
and octopus dreaming
of starfishing above
while humorons try to
remember to love
in a world that nurtures
and cradles all needs
we suckle her dry
then cry on her knee
sweet children of earth
searching for stars
universal expansion
starts within hearts
the first step for all kind
was not on the moon
but at the foot of a friend
who tended a wound
simply by feeling, minding, doing
Empathy is our best
way to human

Growing Up

Stephanie Roche

Growing up, football was my only real passion. It was the one thing that I truly loved and stuck at, through good times and bad. I grew up in a council estate in Shankill, Dublin. Although things weren't always easy, I couldn't have picked a better place to be raised. I learned so much, from how to be tough on the pitch to also having a thick skin off it. Myself and my friends were constantly playing football, we were lucky to have so many different areas to play our matches. We had the main football pitch where Valeview Shankill played, directly in the middle of our estate, an open field outside my house, we also had goalpost painted onto two walls across a road where we played street football and another patch of grass where we played around the block with jumpers for goalposts. It was a young footballers dream.

I saw a lot growing up, the majority of young people around our estate were good people. Some unfortunately just had no focus and that meant they were easily distracted and got involved in other things. Things like drugs, drinking and just getting up to no good in general but for me and my group of friends, we had football. When I look back at my childhood, I always remember it fondly. The group we had, all had their own issues, some parents had a bad relationship with drink, some coming from broken families, some you never knew their issues, but just knew that things weren't always rosy at home and in fairness, there were some who seemed to have a very happy family life. No matter what was going on at home though, we all looked out for each other and made sure we forgot about everything else happening around us, mainly by kicking a ball around from morning 'til night. I think that's the magic of football, even today, I could be having the worst week but when I step onto that pitch, it's all forgotten. For 90+ minutes at least!!

I owe a lot to the people I grew up with and I've never actually told them that, but having the group of friends I did as a kid, helped me become the person I am today. When I see some of the people that grew up in my estate and the direction their lives went, I do think things could have been a lot different for me. That can be put down to making the right decisions at different times but also having a focus. Having a focus as a child is hugely important and our focus was football. The passion and determination I had for the sport was driven a lot by that group of friends. And for that I'm very thankful. I owe a lot to my family also. They have always encouraged me with my football and that was a huge help. My Mam and Dad separated when I was quite young and although it was tough for them both and for us all as a family, they always did their best to ensure that myself, my sister and two brothers were brought up the right way. I was always thought to respect people, no matter who they were or what they did for a living. Respect them. For me, that was respecting the school cleaning lady as much as I would the principal.

I think having the ability to empathise with someone is an ability that not many have, but for me, growing up where I did, I developed that ability from a very young age. And when I became a professional footballer, just like learning to have respect for others, understanding what others were going through and seeing things from their point of view was something that I had to do very often. Sometimes unfortunately, in a team environment, that respect and empathy isn't always reciprocated and that is something that you just have to accept but I always tried to remain respectful and have some degree of empathy towards my teammates and those around me.

From a very young age, I knew I wanted a career in football. However, women's football wasn't as popular as the men's game so for large periods of my childhood, I dreamt of playing for Manchester United alongside Van Nistelrooy and Cole and for Ireland alongside Keane, Duff and Quinn! Being a young girl, playing football, you often heard remarks like 'she shouldn't be playing with the boys', 'she will get hurt playing with them' or 'Look! They have a girl playing for them!' Comments like that were never nice to hear, but I've always been very stubborn and thrived on proving people like that wrong! The dream of playing alongside Keane, Duff, Quinn and co. came to an end when my Dad brought me to my first Irish Women's international match at Richmond Park when I was around twelve. From that day on, I was determined to be the next Olivia O'Toole. What a player, not only was she a woman like me, she was left footed like me too! That was when my journey towards international football began. I had my very first female football role model.

At the age of thirteen, I had trials for the Irish school's team, I got through the first round of trials but unfortunately, I wasn't picked and I was devastated. Not long after, I was asked to trials for Ireland U-17s and it couldn't have gone better. I scored four goals in a training match and the coach rang my Dad to tell him I was picked and just like that, my dream was back on track. I played at both U-17 and U-19s level before finally making my senior debut in 2008. During my time involved in the underage international system, I played with some excellent players. Some who went on to play at senior level with me and some who fell away from the game. Some don't play at all anymore, some maybe felt they were treated badly at times by different coaches and just play club football, I had moments where I thought coaches could have dealt with situations better. But that, unfortunately is the nature of competitive sports, sometimes a player's feelings aren't at the forefront of a coach's mind. For me, the best coaches and managers I had, were the ones who took the time to treat every player with respect and realised that the bad news they were giving us as young players could either make or break us. Too few managers had that thought process though and because of that, a lot of talent got away.

I've been lucky to experience some amazing highs in my career but I've also had some low points. Going from feeling unstoppable, highest of the high to feeling you're not good enough and questioning your ability. They're the emotions you hit as a professional athlete. Being nominated for the Puskas award and attending the Balon D'or awards was a huge high in my career, I had positive comments and high praise from some of the best footballers in the world and I was on cloud nine. My goal was being compared to some of the greatest goals scored in world football and I felt I could do no wrong. Roll on a few years later, a broken leg, some bad moves to clubs that promised me the sun moon and stars when I signed, to them then not paying me (an act extremely unprofessional), and then I'm considered a bad player by some. My point being, some people don't know what is happening or what you go through behind the scenes, it's the highlight reels they want to see and when those highlight reels don't contain wonder goals – you're no longer considered 'a good player'.

I'm extremely proud of my career so far, over fifty caps for Ireland, I've played in some of the best leagues in the world and although I've had some bad experience in recent years, I'm happy to say my love for the game is as big now in my early thirties as it was in my early teens. Although there will always be critics ready to point out your faults and failures, it's the people close to you that remind you of all the great times and remind you that you're career has had more highs than lows. Learning to empathise with my friends and their different circumstances and collectively as a group helping and supporting each other through difficult life experiences when we were kids helped me lay the foundations for which I've built my professional career on. I have carried that ability to empathise with people on my journey whether it be with teammates, rivals, coaches or fans. I feel this has made me a better person, player and teammate throughout my career.

Radiant Empathy in the Dark

Dedicated to Niamh

Ella Anderson

When I was fifteen-years-old, I met someone who changed my life for the better. At that age, I felt depressed and helpless. I had lost all my friends and moved to another school where I knew no one. Although I moved, the pain travelled with me as posts and messages were sent online about me. People I had once seen as friends, slowly disappeared into memories and loneliness overtook, my care for both myself and others lessening. At that age, a lot of people can be oblivious to the effects of their words, especially with cyber bullying allowing a detachment from their actions, sending harmful messages at the touch of a button. A few decades ago, your home would serve as a sanctuary from the abuse you would face at school, but these days it trails behind you everywhere you go.

Such deep feelings of sadness can overtake every aspect of your life – from not brushing your hair properly to not having the energy to shower. When you feel depressed to that level, it's difficult to give yourself basic care because you feel undeserving. If others didn't think you were worth talking to, why would you care for yourself? Having such a lack of self-empathy can make it difficult to empathise with others. You're trapped in a bubble of negative emotion, and the ability to recognise your own feelings and acknowledge them is even more difficult. Although empathy can be learned and strengthened upon, it can also be lost if not practised towards yourself and others.

My friend helped me to change the way I treated myself, and in turn helped me to become more empathetic.

Denying yourself empathy can leave a physical heaviness that weighs you from completing everyday tasks. It shadows you constantly resulting in aspects of your life that are important like education, taking a back seat. Recently, people have become more observant of negative behaviours that mirror depression, but this neglect can be met with disregard. Apathy replaces empathy, providing a shield between you, collecting many more negative emotions, but apathy crowds everything you do. Apathy towards your education, and towards your future. Due to the loss of my friends, I felt apathetic towards all aspects of my life, barely sleeping more than four hours a night. I started to fall asleep in the middle of class, and automatically responded 'I'm fine' when people wanted to know how I was feeling.

I hated myself because I believed everyone else hated me and changing who I was, and my situation, seemed impossible. It was only when I reached my lowest point and experienced such genuine empathy that my mindset started to change. One night when I was fifteen, an online post was written speaking of how terrible a friend I was. It cemented everything I had previously thought about myself, and the weight in my chest sunk to an unknown depth. Luckily, my neighbour had also seen the post and rushed over late in the night to make sure I was okay. Although I had never explicitly said how much I was hurting, she could tell I was not okay. She came into my room in the dead of night, asked me if I was okay and hugged me as I cried in her arms for what felt like minutes, but was hours.

She was and still is the strongest person I have ever known. She carries empathy and compassion in abundance towards everyone. No matter what is thrown at her, she gets back up and it's not for herself – but to make sure that those around her are okay. She witnesses every situation from other perspectives and always refrains from judgement. She recognised my feelings, and I knew that. She is the reason I am who I am and here today. I have never heard her utter a negative comment about anyone, and even if she's put in a situation where nothing is positive, she will find a compliment. You could serve her burnt toast and she would thank you for it. Her empathy fills a room when she walks in, and you can talk to her without judgement. She emphasises in everyday life that no matter how a person may act towards you, you cannot possibly know what's going on in their life and therefore you shouldn't judge them for their actions.

Having someone expressing empathy and being able to recognise when it's necessary to do so in your life, helps you to understand empathy and become more empathetic. Her empathy makes me reflect on my own judgements and allows me to think from another person's perspective. It took her empathy to free me from a cage where I couldn't feel anything but negative emotions. Learning empathy from a perspective of someone with such understanding and care has helped me to understand that we can only control our own actions, and the actions of others may not have been done to intentionally cause harm to you. That person may be hurting too, and they haven't thought about how their actions come across. Allowing that level of understanding between a person and their actions is the key to withholding judgement and building empathy. We don't know what's going on in someone's life, nor do we know how they are feeling and it's important to practise empathy towards everyone, even if they may not do the same to you. Practising empathy towards everyone you meet can only lead to better outcomes.

Learning to be more empathetic has allowed me to understand my own feelings better. We live in such fear of judgement, and sometimes taking a step back and thinking about how we feel can lead to feeling more confident in ourselves. It's okay not to be okay and when I was fifteen, I wasn't. It was receiving an empathetic response that altered my whole perspective. The empathy my best friend expressed, allowed me to think past the boundaries I had made for myself and start to see how she saw me.

Being empathetic towards everyone, even someone you don't know can make a massive difference to that person's world and how they may see themselves. Empathy helps create deeper friendships and greater understanding, resulting in a positive mindset. Now more than ever, in a world where words can be misconstrued so easily, recognising emotion, and expressing empathy can be more difficult than ever. We can hide our emotions through a screen, detach ourselves from our words, and express ourselves in a way that can be perceived differently to how we meant it. Our actions can affect someone deeply, and due to our detachment from our actions we can be blissfully unaware of the pain someone is going through.

Sympathy is seeing someone's pain, whereas empathy is relating and feeling it. I wish I was taught more about empathy when I was younger, and how necessary it is. I wanted to fall in love again with the feeling of being alive, and once I could feel empathy towards myself, empathising with others became easier. By caring for yourself and showing yourself empathy, you can do the same for others. I aspire to be like my best friend.

Empathy and Me

Ashling Dunphy

Some may have called me an angry teenager with a mission of saving the world, others perhaps may have sighed 'notions' under their breath but really I was just doing what I felt was the right thing to do. I can't explain my moral compass but it's my whole being.

I tend to give to others, more than I give to myself but not in any expectancy to receive it back ever. I grew up with the belief that if you don't have enough to share then don't have it at all and I suppose it's gotten me this far.

In 2015 Storm Frank caused a huge amount of damage to housing across the town of Carrick-on-Suir, I, a mouthy sixteen-year-old, took it upon myself to take to Facebook and gather a group of young people to aid the community in their cleaning of the area. Soon christened 'Angels in Wellies' by one of the locals we kept going for almost two weeks. We cleaned houses and garage's before turning our hands to cooking meals for those living alone. We provided food parcels with donations from the local supermarkets and the generous members of the community. We worked together with members of the Carrick-on-Suir River Rescue and Foróige Neighbourhood Youth Projects leaders and young people. Everyday we got up, put on our wellies and waited to be greeted by whatever that day had in store, be it emotional residents upset about the devastation caused in their homes or filling skips with damaged furniture we did it, but most importantly we were there for people. We sat and listened to stories about everything from what was on the morning paper to children and grandchildren who had emigrated to lands far away.

I'm now twenty year's old and whilst I may not be as mouthy and out there as I was when I was sixteen, I believe it is our duty to help and support our fellow members of society. It does not have to be significant but it may make somebody's day, week or even year.

There are always injustices to be tackled, be that locally, nationally or internationally and as a society made up of individuals we can always make somebody's day a little easier. Every job I've worked in, be it on supermarket tills, sweeping and mopping restaurant floors or stacking pallets in a warehouse, one thing I have become aware of is everyone has a story. A story they wish to tell to many, we just need to listen more, not listen to answer but actually stop for a moment, stand back and listen to listen, that person is telling you for a reason and we can learn so much from others.

We need to stop making assumptions about those around us, and the lives they live.

So my advice is simple, Empathy is not complicated. It is a gentle hello and a reassuring smile. Tip the waiter if you can, give a smoke to the lonesome soul, drop a coin in someone's cup, help the lady with the pram getting on the train, cheer on the busker, crack a joke with the gentleman sitting alone on the bus, say thank you to the taxi driver, and always stand up for the underdog.

You don't know what has happened in the hours or years before you came across that person. That somebody may be mourning a loss, facing homelessness, waiting on medical results, trying to further their education, braving the wave of mental health or just having a bad day.

It's not about the money, cigarette or recognition. It's about silently going about your day recognising that as human beings our lives are severely complicated and whilst we are aware that everyday may not be a good day, something good happens everyday.

Rest assured that when you're having a bad day someone else will return the favour and loan you their smile.

Think a little before you judge anyone else's livelihood or circumstances.

Thank you to all who took part and helped 'Angels and Wellies' help others.

Broken Radios

Fiona Prine

I stood pinned to the damp wall at the back of the National Boxing Stadium in Dublin. It was 1979 and my boyfriend had given me two tickets to see John Prine in concert. My friend and I had no idea who this kind-of-funny-looking American Folk singer was, and we didn't have much connection to his songs, or his three-piece band.

At that time, we were fans of the likes of Leonard Cohen, Lou Reed, Van Morrison, Cat Stevens and Thin Lizzy. I listened to female writers and would try to imagine myself in some of their lyrics – Joni Mitchell, Janis Ian, Carol King. This was different. I remember John sang story songs about people but about American people whose lives were so, so, different from my own, train-wrecked, life. Little did I know …

My friend and I stood to leave our seats mid-way through the concert and made our way to the back of the venue. We stood there, of course, until the song was finished, before making our getaway. And that is when I recognised Empathy for the very first time in my life; at a time when I needed a sign from somewhere that I was still in touch with reality, that everything was OK when all seemed eschew and chaotic around me. I was a teenager, struggling emotionally, trying to make sense of my life.

The song was Sam Stone, and the line was, '… Sweet songs never last too long on broken radios …'

It burned right through the protective shell I had built around my shame, hurt, loneliness and grief.

I felt my gut churn and tears stung the corners of my eyes. Who WAS this fella? And how could he possibly know that all the sweet songs in my life had evaporated and that the radio had been silenced? I know it was my very first true experience with empathy and it turned out to be an experience that would prove to be life-changing in every possible way.

Growing up in rural Ireland of the 1960s and 1970s was, in many ways, not a hospitable place for a child. Only now do we know, and are continuing to learn about, the full extent of the abuse of power perpetrated by the Catholic church the mother and baby homes, Magdalene laundries, clerical sexual abuse, so called corporal punishment in schools, and of course the Children Should Be Seen and not Heard guidance about child-rearing inflicted on God-fearing parents. Northern Ireland was in turmoil with The Troubles sometimes spilling over to south of the border.

On 22 March 1975, my father was killed in a headlong collision with a large vehicle on the road home from a teacher's conference in the south of Ireland.

We lived in Ardara, Co. Donegal, the lovely village where my parents were born and where I was raised along with my five younger sisters. To say that my father's death was a traumatic tragedy is so much of an understatement. He was the headmaster of our local National School, an involved and active member of our small community, and a trusted advisor and mentor admired by all who knew and loved him. For me, and my mother and sisters, it might just have been that the large vehicle had driven through the centre of our home that day. Donal Whelan had been my Daddy but had also been my teacher from age three when I went to school with him, probably to alleviate the burden on my mother who by that time had other babies to care for.

There was no talk at that time of counselling or of emotional help with the enormity of what had happened to our family. We were encouraged to 'get on with it' and ultimately, that is what we did. My mother had to work now, finding herself the single parent and sole provider of six young daughters. Within a year of his death, she made the decision to move us to Dublin. At the time, it seemed impossible, brave, or downright crazy – depending on who was offering the unsolicited opinion, and there were many. But move we did – on my fourteenth birthday, 4 August 1975. I can still remember being driven out of the village, stunned by a mixture of sadness, excitement and fear. Those early years were hard. They were hard for all of us in similar and in different ways. But we survived and ultimately thrived – though that took some time.

I remember after my father's death having the strongest conviction that since THAT had happened – that I had lost the first man who truly loved me, the one who saw my intelligence, my creative sensibilities and talent, and had, kindly remarked on my blossoming girlhood as I entered my teenage years, that just about ANYTHING could happen to me in the times ahead. I was aware that there could be danger, loss, pain and challenges, but that there could maybe, just maybe, be fantastical wonder and joy. After all, the most unbelievable thing had happened – who knew what else Life had in store for me?

That night in The Stadium I felt empathy flowing from a man I did not know and had no idea that I ever would know …

That first decade in Dublin did indeed present many challenges. I finished my education, worked, and gave birth to my oldest son – a gift beyond measure for me at that time, and to this day. But I was still searching for that feeling from that one person. Someone who would see me and hear me and recognise a well bruised but tender heart, a bright and curious mind, and a generous empathic spirit behind the breezy and steely exterior.

I worked at Windmill Lane Studios in the late 1980s and attended both opening nights of the nearby, Point Depot now known as The 3Arena in November 1988.

The music roster both nights was filled with artists we would now regard as part of the Americana/Roots genre – Everly Brothers, Lyle Lovett, Joe Ely, Flaco Jimenez, Guy Clark, Cowboy Jack Clement and the one artist who would later earn the accolade of the Godfather of Americana, my beloved and so sorely missed late husband, John Prine.

We met at a raucous after-party in Blooms Hotel on 28 November 1988. My high school friend, and well-respected Blues singer, Mary Stokes, introduced us. Although it would be several years later that we would marry and together grow a family, that spark of empathy was undoubtedly there from the minute we met. I recognised it immediately.

John had always assumed, as a human being and as an artist, that there was pain and hurt and happiness and joy in everybody's life story. He accepted people, and if he loved you, he loved you unconditionally. He understood the void that deep loss can leave inside and he believed that we all have a capacity for love, regardless of our circumstances and choices. And John Prine believed in magic – that just about anything can and does happen in this one wild life we are given. I agree.

I truly believe that empathy can and must be taught; empathy must be SHOWN to our children. Empathy is tangible and real; it is the feeling of understanding, appreciation, respect and connection and it can be taught and demonstrated in so many ways – through music, song, poetry, dance, talking and listening, paintings, film, letter writing …

More than anything else I believe with all my heart that children must be Seen and Heard if they are to grow to become empathic adults who can dream and dare to be all they can be.

Ingredients

Neven Maguire

'When you give you get' was something my mother used to say. And if you love food you will never be short of opportunities to give some pleasure, whether by feeding people, or teaching them to cook. I always think of cooking as an essential life skill.

My mother and father were steeped in the hospitality industry. They first opened the MacNean Restaurant. They kept the business going throughout the toughest of times. Bomb scares and actual explosions were a feature of life in Blacklion. We are right on the border and there were times that the business was just not viable and they had nine children to raise. During one of those closures, my dad opened a restaurant in Sligo and sadly it was on his way to that restaurant one night that he lost his life in a motor accident. I was in my first season of cooking each Tuesday afternoon on *Open House* with Mary & Marty and he had driven me to the studio each week and was very proud of how it was going. My parents gave all of their children a great start in life. It was drilled into us that every customer is out for a special meal and it is up to us to make that as good an experience as possible.

When times improved my mum opened the restaurant again on her own, with me to help. Eventually I took over, by then they had laid the foundations, and she was there for much needed advice for many more years. No one does this job unless they love it and you have to love people also. Plus you have to believe in people. And they did. They loved giving young people a chance and encouraging them.

I was the first boy to do Home Economics at Fermanagh Catering College. I might have got a bit of teasing, but nothing much. And I couldn't have cared less. It was what I wanted to do. I had a wonderful teacher, Mairead McMorrow, and she gave me a great foundation. My parents opened my eyes to the world that was out there and made sure I trained in good European restaurants, with Lea Linster in Luxembourg and Arzac in the Basque county among them. I think they would both be happy that Blacklion has remained at the centre of my life and that this is where Amelda and I decided to raise our family. I think they would also be glad that we have a kitchen where there is no shouting and screaming. I am surrounded by a fantastic team of people who are very good at what they do and love doing it.

The restaurant and kitchen are in my blood, but I have been surprised by how much enjoyment I have had doing demos. People are so willing, even eager, to learn. Despite being in the hospitality business it is my mission for more and more people to enjoy cooking good Irish produce at home. Doing demos is like a tonic, and I was surprised during all of the lockdowns that they are almost as good on ZOOM. Also, we did some that would not have been possible face to face. Before Christmas, I had two great sessions with staff who work in our embassies. They weren't able to get home for Christmas and it was like having another two Christmas parties. Cooking has brought me so many great opportunities.

There is another group of budding cooks who stick in my mind. I was asked by the National Council for the Blind in Ireland to put on some demos. I learned so much by doing them. It forced me to be really clear about what I was doing and saying. I was fascinated by the kitchen gadgets that had been adapted for their particular needs. I have done a few of these sessions now and I really look forward to them. Believe it or not, we did one on ZOOM and I think we were all delighted with how it worked out.

Social media forms an increasing part of my world. I have been fortunate but I do find it sad how many people are cruel about all sorts of things on the various platforms. Writing nasty things about a restaurant that can be totally unfounded can damage business. And how much worse if it is about a person. The worst I have to deal with are people who give out about my accent or some of the phrases I use on my TV programmes which do not come up to their particular standards for the English language. I feel sorry for such people who have not been lucky enough to live in Cavan! The positive side of social media is brilliant. A compliment goes a long way.

I was delighted to be asked to contribute some thoughts to this book. It took a little time to think about but time is one of the things I learned a lot about during Covid. Time with people you love is very special and I relearned to appreciate it during 2020 – I won't be giving it up again easily. Family time is special and it is one of those true clichés that children grow up very quickly.

I have been very lucky. I have been able to turn my passion into my job. As I reminded people when I rediscovered my decks, dance music was also a passion. Thankfully I had the common sense to see which passion to keep as a hobby and which to pursue! With the decks I may have been more enthusiastic than talented! If you love your job it doesn't feel like work. If you are enjoying your work, and indeed life in general, you are kinder to other people and happy to give them the opportunity to develop their skills and talents. I have loved seeing the great chefs in our kitchen develop and often go on to other things. Plenty of people gave me a leg up when I needed it. It is not hard to give a little back. And as my mother would have said, 'it feels surprisingly good'.

He Fell through the Cracks

Rita Ann Higgins

The boy's name was Abel.
At times he was sunny,
oftener he was sad.
He was non-verbal himself –
the voices in his head
like a Greek chorus,
never took a tea break.

He couldn't tell you what they said.
He went around the house
with his hands covering his ears
trying to block out the hub-bub.

His mother cried the day the van came.
They put him in an adult Psych ward.
He shared the ward with four men
who had their own demons.
They never got a weekend pass,
much less a visitor with some smokes.

Abel deteriorated,
his mother told doctors.
A flock of them around his bed.
The white swans of Coole.
What's wrong love, she'd say.
He couldn't tell her what toy he wanted.
His remote-control dinosaur, his Ninja set!

She guessed on and on for a solid week.
Every toy he owned was named, some twice over.
He slid into the quieter rooms in his head.
He didn't cover his ears anymore.

When his file was analysed,
the professionals said,
Abel fell through the cracks.

He went in in a van,
a jalopy of a thing.
He came home in a box,
a pencil case of a thing.

Citylink Tales

Catherine Denning

I sat beside Nigel, a homeless man, today

I lie

For the last five days a portaloo
has been his home in Salthill, County Galway

He has kind eyes

They glowed when he spoke of the site worker
Who afforded him a few extra hours sleep on a torrential
    September morning
On our Wild Atlantic Way

They sparkled when he related how that same kind worker
Removed only the neighbouring loo
To gift Nigel an extra day in his chemical shelter from the
    storm

It gets fierce wet in the west, in fairness

As an adjunct
He gleams at his use of a pilfered 'Out of Order' sign
That he used to don his home's front door
To deter the longing and urgent passers by

And took pleasure from running the needy college fresher

Who begged to do his unmerciful business in Nigel's not so
porcelain bowl

Nigel lacked some empathy there,
With my granted understanding

Nigel regaled me with tales of Maeve
Twenty years his junior
Who was drinking herself into an early grave

Seizures, missing person's lists
He calls hospitals and shelters
It keeps him, daily, sustained

Does empathy have borders
Who am I to know?

He tells me of sneaking in to charge his phone in the
aquarium
The lonely fish in their containers there
Not supposed to be fitted in.

Thinking in Plastic

Ciara-Beth Ní Ghríofa

My favourite thing about the human brain, is that we describe it as being plastic. The networks and pathways within our brains are constantly changing and adapting based on our lived experiences. It means that as individuals, we're capable of change. If we want to change how we speak, or how we interact with people, or act to correct our own biases, we can. With limited exceptions, most humans are capable of changing their behaviour. Which means, most humans, have the ability to learn empathy.

It seems to me, that learning empathy is similar to learning to speak. Most people are born with the capacity to learn to speak, but can't do so without being exposed to language. In most cases, as a child becomes exposed to more complex language, they start to string words together to form sentences, and their vocabulary becomes richer. Similarly, most of us are born with the capacity to learn empathy, but unless we're exposed to empathetic behaviour, we don't have the opportunity to expand on our ability to empathise.

As such, getting empathy into our classrooms isn't just a matter of adding it to the curriculum and preaching to students about being empathetic. In order to learn empathy, students need to be shown empathy. As young people, we're often told that we're being melodramatic when we're upset about a problem we have, or that 'life's not fair' when we share our thoughts about an inequality we're dealing with. In my experience, it has been rare that an adult authority figure would sit with me and acknowledge my feelings if I was upset or angry. All too often, they'd talk about how life is hard, and that your teenage years are the best years of your life, and tell me that I'd have much bigger problems to deal with in the real world. Don't get me wrong, these adults meant well, but the end result was that I'd always feel like I wasn't being listened to, on top of all of the problems I was already experiencing. Can we really expect children and teenagers to show empathy if we're not willing to show them what empathy looks like?

As an autistic person, I've spent the first twenty-one years of my life being taught how to make my autism less obvious to those around me. Autism treatment frequently focuses on teaching us how to 'mask', to make it seem like we're neuro-typical. Masking is an exhausting process, but is one that we're taught from an early age is necessary. I'm of the opinion that our society needs to learn to be more empathetic to people who are different. Instead of teaching autistic people tricks to make it seem like we're neurotypical, we should be teaching people why autistic people do the things we do, or at the very least teaching that people sometimes look or act differently to how we ourselves act or look, and that it's ok.

So many negative experiences that I had as a teenager could have been so different if the people involved had shown some empathy. Instead of learning to think about how our actions affect other people, we're taught not to do or say anything that might make us a target for bullies. Now as a young adult, I'm being told that workplaces are striving for diversity and inclusion, and that it's ok to be different, but how can we have diverse and inclusive workplaces when we're telling young people that they should actively try to make the very traits that make them diverse less obvious?

Additionally, if we're genuinely trying to make workplaces

more diverse and inclusive, empathy is going to play a critical role in fostering an inclusive environment. Without empathy and understanding, it will prove difficult if not impossible to make a work environment truly accessible to neurodiverse individuals. Many workplaces have recently started 'autism-friendly hiring' initiatives, which frequently involve making accommodations to the interview process, and it's fantastic to see businesses that are enthusiastic about including those of us who aren't neurotypical, but my concern is that unless these accommodations are being implemented with a proper understanding as to why they're necessary, they may not actually be as helpful as they appear on the surface. Unless you're also willing to offer similar accommodations to the individual if they're hired, it might be more challenging for us to succeed in your workplace. Sometimes neurotypical people forget to apply empathy to a situation, and they believe that accommodations such as allowing an autistic employee to use headphones, or allowing them to take more frequent short breaks, are giving an unfair advantage in some way. When looking at the same situation with empathy, it becomes apparent that autistic people perceive the world in a completely different way, and those accommodations are likely making it possible for us to do our job.

Even outside of employment, empathy is a major factor in how accessible I find spaces such as shops, museums, restaurants and similar spaces. Being able to return at a given time instead of waiting in a queue that would put me into sensory overload, or being permitted to keep my backpack which helps me regulate my sensory system, or having staff understand that even though I'm wearing headphones to block out sound in a noisy restaurant that I'm still able to hear them, can be the difference in being able to stay and enjoy myself and feeling miserable to the point where I have to leave. A little bit of empathy costs nothing, but can make the world more accessible to people like me.

So even though the world is chaotic, life gets busy, and you probably have loads on your mind already, the pathways in your brains are constantly changing, and the choice is yours: will you practise empathy?

Courageous Conversations

On a Friday Evening can Change your Life

Fr Ben Hughes

There's Something about a Friday Evening

It is a Friday evening at 4.30 p.m. and the university lecture halls have emptied and the car parks are vacated. The university campus has become quiet as staff and students have packed their bags and have retreated home for the weekend. A call comes through on our student support helpline and it is a student's voice hesitantly asking if there is someone they could meet to talk with for a few minutes. We make arrangements to meet on campus at 5.00 p.m. As the conversation begins the issue seems normal and manageable. The student is looking for advice about how best to manage an argument that they had with a friend. Forty minutes later, the complexity of the story is beginning to emerge.

The argument with the friend happened because the friend is concerned about this student's behaviour. Having acknowledged that managing arguments with friends who challenge our behaviour is difficult, the student began to speak more quietly, the eye contact lessens and there a small cough before the tears begin to fall. They somehow realise that they are now telling the precious story of their life. Perhaps they are not so aware that this is a significant turning point in their life that can influence their entire journey. The student apologies for crying and then reassures me that they are really OK as the tears now flow even harder. Having reassured them that they are in the right place and that we will work this through together the student continues to talk.

Fifty minutes later the underlying struggles of this student's story is still unfolding. They explain that they are relying heavily on alcohol and drugs, not attending lectures and feeling lonely. While they are passing exams and connecting with friends, at a surface level, they feel lost and are not comfortable in themselves. As they continue to talk, the conversation now includes stories about their growing up days at home, experiences of secondary school and the challenges of university life.

The argument with a friend has triggered an existential moment which has motivated this student to reach out and courageously ask for help. The meeting ends with the reassurance of on-going support which happens over next few weeks. During those weeks the student gains new insights, understands how their problematic behaviours had slowly emerged and the purpose they were serving. Their desire is to let go of the behaviours that are no longer working and to develop new life-giving ways of engaging with the world. The power of an empathic conversation allowed their heart to open, and as the tears fell the healing began. Having the wisdom to have a courageous conversation on any evening can change the rest of your life, for the better.

The Background Context

The University of Galway is where the Friday evening conversation took place. The University of Galway is located in the city of Galway in the West of Ireland, along the Wild Atlantic Way. Galway city, affectionately known as the City of the Tribes, is renowned as a city of culture and diversity. This diversity is particularly complemented by the vibrancy and creativity of a population of over 18,000 students making

Galway their home for the duration of their studies. The Friday evening conversation reflects the many sacred stories that are told in the context of my work in the department of Student Support Services as pastoral counsellor.

In this work I am continually grateful to experience the joys and sorrows of our students who aim high, achieve much and reach out to realise their full potential. It is truly energising to be surrounded by students who are striving, dreaming, creating, discerning and reflecting on life. It is amazing to witness how discipline is honed, challenge is embraced, and high performance is achieved within our university community. As a psychotherapist, it is equally satisfying to support students in overcoming obstacles, developing tenacity and becoming resilient. As a pastor, it is soulful to witness the deep generosity of our students and staff who are compassionate, kind and empathetic by nature. It is similarly gratifying to work with so many colleagues who continuously strive to provide opportunities for students to enhance their personal wellbeing, expand tolerance and inspire innovation. The university staff are excellent at awakening creativity, igniting curiosity and creating pathways for our students to become their best selves. The staff provide such support with the intention of helping students realise their goals. This support is undertaken in the hope that the students will experience happiness and success as the journey of their precious lives unfold.

The Inevitable Challenges of Life

In the midst of all the positive engagement that embodies our leafy green campus, students experience the inevitable challenges of life. These challenges sometimes generate anxiety and confusion. Thankfully, when this happens students can usually dig deep into their own personal and psychological reserves to find what they need to regain their balance. In supporting students who experience such challenges, the university provides a range of supports. These supports frequently provide a valuable stepping-stone towards navigating the difficult experience. Difficulties are never easy; in many instances, though they become a learning opportunity, that facilitates a student to gain new insight. It is heartening to see students learn how to resolve their dilemmas, recalibrate their emotions and successfully move forward. While many students successfully manage to negotiate the difficult situations and emotions that they encounter, there are some for whom these difficulties become complex, prolonged and unmanageable. In some instances, the situation may generate feelings of hopelessness and despair.

Dark Days

In 2014, the sense of students' hopelessness was observed in a dramatic rise in accidental and suicidal deaths in the Galway area among young people. The suddenness of these unexpected deaths created a wave of sadness and grief for the University of Galway Community. Naturally, it caused great pain and suffering to students, their families and friends. This sense of pain and loss was also experienced among our staff who worked with these young people. The lives of those students who died were lovingly remembered at our memorial services on campus and their names are inscribed in the memorial garden at the heart of the university campus. In the aftermath of this immense sadness, we, as a university community, pondered about how best we could respond and initiatives we could take to prevent this kind of loss and suffering.

Empathic Response

In response to these unexpected deaths, a group of staff and students gathered to explore the actions they could take to support students who feel overwhelmed. The group included representatives from the Students Union, the Student Support Services and the Chaplaincy. At our gathering, students talked about the concerns that were causing them anxiety or a sense of hopelessness. The big issues that emerged include mental health, suicide, substance use, relationships and sexuality, finance, family and, of course, academic challenges. As our conversations unfolded, students explained that at times their coping mechanisms are not as robust as they would like in dealing with the inevitable challenges that they experience. Their fragile coping skills result in low tolerance levels to manage their challenges. Students explained that they often lacked knowledge and information about the difficulties experienced. From their experience students said that there was a scarcity of supports and that access to support was overly complex and prohibitive. These obstacles were some of the triggers that pushed students towards hopelessness. These obstacles negatively impacted the student's personal life, their engagement and progression in the university. The group of students and staff who gathered, committed themselves to pursuing a solution to address the key concerns identified by students, and the chaplaincy took responsibility to explore potential solutions.

The exploration began with an investigation of the programmes that were in existence in Ireland, the UK and the United States of America to address similar issues among a university population. While there were several programmes, none had the capacity to translate easily in the University of Galway context. Although disappointing, the absence of a programme that would address the needs of the university community led to the development of a tailored support system to address the issues experienced by the students. This new programme has become a welcome addition to the menu of supports that are already in place and is called 'Seas Suas'.

A New Programme of Support is Born

Seas Suas are Irish words meaning 'Stand Up'. The key objectives of the programme are to motivate students to be more aware and observant of challenging issues impacting students' lives and to equip students with the knowledge and skills to respond appropriately. The Seas Suas programme provides information and training in relation to the concerns identified by students including mental health, substance use, relationships and suicide prevention. The programme is sufficiently flexible to respond to any organically emerging issues. While the programme explicitly addresses specific challenging concerns faced by students, the character of the programme is holistic with a strong focus on health and well-being. In doing so, Seas Suas aims to foster a culture of care and support within the University of Galway community and beyond by promoting positive well-being, empathy, skilled intervention, and a pro-social attitude. The theoretical model that underpins the programme is Darley and Latané's (1968) Bystander Intervention Model and the Life Skills Programme in the University of Arizona . The Seas Suas programme began in autumn 2014 with forty-five students. Since 2016, 500 students' volunteers are trained each year and the demand for the programme consistently exceeds capacity.

Holistic and Interactive Training

Students undertaking the Seas Suas training attend four consecutive two-hour training sessions, and afterwards complete a reflective journal exercise. Each training session focuses on a different topic, facilitated by a leading expert in that field. In these training sessions, students are provided with information about challenging student issues and the corresponding supports. Students are asked to reflect on the concerns, develop strategies for effective helping, and in this way students build new skills in safe intervention and referral. Each training session includes interactive engagement, reflective practice and opportunities for a practical application of their learning. After training, students are encouraged to put their learning into action in a variety of ways. Over the years, students contribute to a number of relevant campaigns such as the 'Mental Health Green Ribbon' campaign, and the 'Darkness into Light' campaign for suicide prevention. Together with the University Examination Support Team, Seas Suas volunteers provide peer-mentoring to students. The Seas Suas programme is organised in collaboration with the UNESCO Child and Family Research Centre at the University of Galway and collaborates with a host of external stakeholders including Mental Health Ireland, the National Office for Suicide Prevention, the Western Region Drug and Alcohol Task Force, and the Samaritans.

Out of Darkness a Light Has Shone

Since the dark days of 2014 when we mourned the sad loss of too many of our young people the Seas Suas programme has become a beacon of light. It has unlocked the opportunity for student participants to express empathy and kindness to those in need of support. We hear of, and witness, countless instances where students who have completed the programme become the Good Samaritan and successfully undertake a compassionate intervention. These skilled interventions help those in need to successfully manage difficult situations and emotions. Such interventions are all the more poignant when the issues are complex, prolonged and difficult to manage. In cultivating and generating empathy the Seas Suas programme reduces hopelessness and has been life-saving and life-giving. The programme helps those with difficulties to manage their crises, that otherwise have the potential to overwhelm and lead to despair. The Seas Suas programme equips students to identify supports, provide opportunities for second chances and new beginnings.

In addition to the anecdotal stories that we hear about the positive impact of the programme, we are grateful to our partners in the UNESCO Child and Family Research Centre at the University of Galway for their research on the programme. Research results consistently report that the Seas Suas programme is associated with a number of positive outcomes . In particular, participants show significantly higher levels of empathy, express more positive social responsibility values, and feel more confident in their skills to help and understand others having completed the Seas Suas programme. In addition, respondents appear to believe that participation in the programme is associated with a number of benefits, attributing increases in their knowledge of student issues, awareness of others in need, willingness to help others, and confidence in their ability to intervene as a result of their participation in the Seas Suas programme.

Empathy Works

Empathy is inextricably interwoven into the Seas Suas programme, which is an appealing aspect of the programme. From our personal experiences, we all recognise empathy as something that is highly valuable. In different ways, we all long for experienced and generously given empathy. The consistent aura of empathy in the Seas Suas programme speaks attentively to our human story and reflects our daily experiences. The empathy of Seas Suas ignites something deep within us and serves to both comfort and motivate us.

Seas Suas, in its design and delivery, recognises that life can be challenging and that we can all benefit from having support, particularly when we feel fragile. Consequently, Seas Suas gives students permission to reflect on their own lives, identify issues in need of attention and engage supports that will be helpful. Underpinning all of this is the subtle invitation to cultivate self-empathy and the encouragement to show compassion and kindness to oneself, in the first instance. The key invitation is to have the courage to ask for the help that we need. When we reach out for help, both the magic of life and goodness of the world ensure the answers we seek will come towards us. In addition to developing self-empathy, the programme proactively trains students to deepen their awareness and sensitivity towards helping others. The students' heightened awareness and skills-training become the ideal channel to unlock an abundance of natural empathy. This empathy is then expressed by an outpouring of support and kindness in caring for others and for the environment.

Live Your One Precious Life to the Full

Once the students complete the Seas Suas programme, their achievement is marked with an award ceremony. At that ceremony, students are reminded about the inevitability of difficulties in life and emphasise that difficulties usually do not last forever. They are encouraged to ask for help, and in their own way to remain generous in offering support to others along the journey of life. As they complete the programme, students are reminded that they are only required to take one step at a time, to travel lightly through life and to trust that things will work out. It is explained to them that they are resourceful and that the answers to their difficulties may be closer to them than they think. As the students' generosity is honoured, it is reiterated that their empathy, their idealism and their commitment to justice is making a difference for the better. It is emphasised that such values will open up the pathway towards personal fulfilment, success and happiness for themselves and for others. Finally, the students are reminded that they have one precious life to live and we encourage them to live it to the full.

Conclusion

In a world that is often challenging Seas Suas teaches all of us that the gift of empathy can be the pathway to a sheltering place particularly when life feels stormy and uncertain. Empathy reminds us that the world does care, that life is manageable and that support is available. The Seas Suas programme promotes the belief that empathy is the magic that builds relationships, generates hope and facilitates healing. Empathy reassures us that 'everything will be all right in the end. If it's not all right, then it's not the end'.

My Understanding of Empathy

Timmy Long

I first understood the meaning of empathy in my mid-thirties after nearly twenty years of alcohol and drug addiction. As an addict and alcoholic, one of the main psychological characteristics is the feeling of numbness, emotionally, mentally and spiritually. I was so out of touch with my own feelings and emotions that it was impossible to know what a word like empathy really meant. It is my belief that empathy comes from the association of experiences between people who share similar traumatic experiences, struggles and adversities.

When I see someone going through their daily struggle from addiction, no matter which one, there are two feelings that come to the forefront of my consciousness, and they are empathy and gratitude. For someone like me to see another person in the exact position I was in ten years ago, my heart bleeds for them, and I get an overwhelming feeling of gratitude for my life at present.

Growing up as a young child, our family home was frequently violent and a scary place for any child, poor mental health was also obvious from the outside, looking in. My experiences of these situations still live within my body as feelings of shame, guilt, fear and unworthiness. It is here that the word empathy can be genuinely understood for me, when I see a child living within an environment like mine as a child. The understanding of the word can be fully respected, however, with a heavy heart and a tear to my eye for those that still suffer.

Empathy to Me

James Leonard

Empathy is the mother who always knew how I was feeling,

Empathy is the father who showed me how to paint a ceiling.

Empathy is the teacher who nurtured my love for history,

Empathy is the youth worker who explained some of life's mysteries.

Empathy is the aunt who never judged once the drugs came,

Empathy is my brother's love when all I could feel was shame.

Empathy is the sister who always left the door ajar,

Empathy is the therapist who helped heal emotional scars.

Empathy is the key worker who treated me like a human,

In spite of all the alcohol and drugs I was consuming.

Empathy is paramedics who helped me over the years,

You helped relieve my parents' worries even if they were still in tears.

Empathy is the garda who showed concern and kindness,

When I was walking down the road, stoned, numb and mindless.

Empathy is the treatment centre who helped to change my mindset,

And helped me through the rats, night terrors, sickness and colds sweats.

Empathy is charity that gave me a bed and aftercare,

Empathy is the wife who told me to have no fear.

Empathy is the university that gave me opportunities and knowledge,

You helped make the whole experience amazing in college.

Empathy is the employer who gave me chance in spite of my convictions,

Empathy is my podcast and those who always listen.

Empathy is a life-saver and helped to change the game,

Empathy saved me, it helped to rescue James.

Empathy can Heal our Troubled World

Shaykh Dr Umar Al-Qadri

As a person of faith, I believe faith to be something liberating, something that gives joy in our times of happiness and solace in our times of sorrow. A lack of empathy in religious people – worse, visibly religious people, and worse still, religious leaders or the clergy – has throughout the world turned people away not only from the formal structures and hierarchies of faith (perhaps not a bad thing) but from faith itself.

Because when we think of religious people, empathy definitely isn't the first thing that comes to mind. There's a concept of religious people as harsh, conservative or judgemental. Whether it be in the history of my country, Ireland, and the generations of priests and nuns who limited life opportunities for single mothers, or whether it be in the contemporary troubles of Afghanistan, with the Taliban limiting women's rights in pursuit of supposed religious purity, empathy is definitely not high enough on our collective religious agendas. As a person of faith, a faith leader, indeed, this makes me sad.

All religions in their truest form have empathy at their core. Indeed, so central is empathy to true faith and religion that it has been called 'the golden rule' – be it the 'Love for your brother what you love for yourself' of my faith, Islam, the 'Do unto your neighbour as you would have done unto you' of Christianity or the near identical commandment found in nearly all major and minor religions in the history of the world, there is no faith without empathy.

Gifts and gestures do not always cross linguistic, cultural and theological boundaries and borders well. A simple thumbs up, a seal of approval throughout most of the world, is an offensive gesture in parts of Afghanistan. Candles are a semi-passive form of remembrance and hope in Catholicism, an active form of 'fire-worship' in Hinduism, and yet considered a superfluous extravagance in strands of Protestantism and Islam. Throughout the western world, the bride wears white on her wedding day – in the Indian subcontinent, the Hindu widow wears white to symbolise her grief. You are beginning to understand how difficult it is to find a single, universal gesture of solidarity and compassion, of our siblinghood in the human family, that translates well to all times and places.

It is this universality of empathy that makes it so essential as we navigate our way through this complicated world. Everyone, regardless of their language, background, creed or absence of, or economic status can understand empathy. It is a gift we can confidently give and receive wherever we find ourselves in the world, even when separated by issues of communication and language.

Empathy is universal in other ways too: it need not be an in-person experience – we can feel empathies for individuals whether they are known to us or strangers, friends or enemies. A well-known example from the life of the Prophet Muhammad (peace be upon him) comes to my mind, when he told his companions, 'Assist your brother, the oppressor and the oppressed'. Confused, his companions asked him, 'How do we assist the oppressor?' to which he replied, 'By stopping him'. We can widen this analogy out to our approach to crime and social exclusion in our societies.

There is no doubt that crime and anti-social behaviour causes great harm in our societies. But rather than merely seek to condemn, we can take an empathetic approach, seeking rehabilitative and restorative approaches to justice that make us all safer by preventing crime at its roots, rather than the reactionary calls for ever punishments that cloud our conversations at every level of society, from social media to our political establishments.

We can feel empathy for groups, societies and entire nations too. This is even more important in an age of twenty-four hour news coverage, digital and social media, when constant exposure to tragedy and trauma threatens to desensitise us. At the time of writing, wars have raged in Syria for over ten years, whilst children starve to death in Yemen on a daily basis. The people of Palestine continue to suffer whilst no solution appears obvious. The pandemic appears to be entering its end game in Europe and the developed world, whilst vaccine rollout remains in the single percentage digits in the global south. Whilst the details may change by the year and the decade, this theme remains the same.

Our globalised society is today more interconnected than ever before in human history. As western citizens, we hold an enormous amount of arbitrary and, if we are honest, unfair influence over global policy. A true empathy for those we share our planet with requires ethnical consumption and lobbying of our political establishments. With continued activism and the judicious application of pressure, real and lasting change is possible in our world. From our success in reversing damage to the ozone layer to the end of apartheid in South Africa, our collective empathy has proven its ability to deliver such change.

Let me end, then, with a call to action: let us try to implement three acts of empathy in every day, on any of the levels I have discussed. Personal, societal or international empathy possess the very real power to change our world, to build bridges over divides and to heal our troubled world. We have tried suspicion and hatred, the results litter the pages of the history books. Let's work towards a brighter future with empathy.

Empathy *Sa Chistin*

Therese, Aine, and Aidan Hume

Empathy is a core element of wisdom. It holds the light of kindness to reality, and softens it, seeding acceptance and healing. It can bring joy to the everyday and make the unbearable bearable. In the public realm, it is the foundation for the mutual understanding that precedes peace and informs justice. Tempered by love and compassion, empathetic action builds and maintains the peaceful societies and healthy ecosystems necessary for planetary sustainability and thriving future generations.

The notion of empathy was core to our parents' work and beliefs. Despite his studies for the priesthood, our father emphasised only one line in the bible as being truly important: 'Do unto others as you would have them do unto you', or as alternatively stated: 'love thy neighbour as thyself'. His earlier community involvement was greatly influenced by his childhood experience of overcrowded conditions. He understood well the difficulty of families who lacked the essential security of a decent home. This led to his work in forming the Derry Housing Association. Similarly, his experience of poverty, as his father spent many years unemployed, no doubt shaped his strong belief in the emancipatory role of education. It also led to his involvement with the Credit Union movement and to supporting those trying to establish local businesses to provide jobs. As he observed in a 1964 *[The] Irish Times* article:

> Such community activity, in which all sections play their part can do nothing but create mutual respect and above all, build the

> country with our own hands. It will also water down the deep prejudice which is at the root of discrimination.

This 'blatant discrimination', and the 'deep prejudice which is its cause', were endemic in Northern Ireland at the time, the article noting that 'it is at its point-of-origin prejudice that discrimination should be tackled'. It was the structural inequalities feeding the persistence of this discrimination that would ultimately raise the need for action at a political level, resulting in his involvement in politics. The need for political and social systems that would meet these basic human needs was central to his work.

Central to this political philosophy was the need to understand the psychology and beliefs of others. The political solutions he advocated involved mending and building relationships at different levels as well as acknowledging and accommodating diversity. In a 1979 article in the journal Foreign Affairs, he observed that the: 'protagonists do act in the light of their interests as they perceive them, though their perceptions are sometimes mistaken.' Exploration of the deep fears and insecurities of others can provide hope and the 'possibility of solutions to the most intractable impasses'. In a later speech in 1983, he eschews the need for exclusive access to power, stating that 'any country is richer for diversity', that it 'is not possible permanently to exclude an entire section of the population from any say in the decision-making process', and asking 'What is wrong with asking to be able to build structures whereby the different traditions can live in peace, harmony and unity?'

This political work was highly stressful, but through it he was supported by our mother, Pat, and a broader community of neighbours, party-members and other random individuals who might land at the front door for various reasons. Growing up in 6 West End Park Derry, we would find empathy, often in situations and stories of comedy, between the pulley line, the Aga cooker and the Sacred Heart picture in the tiny kitchen. Somehow, despite the waves of chaos and sorrow which beset those days, there was warmth and humour to sustain us in the many folk who joined us in that kitchen. Molly Doherty, or Nana as we called her, was a constant figure. Our Granny's best friend, she would arrive to see our mother out to work, then mind us until one by one she saw us off to school. Watching our father's deepening preoccupation, she would guide him very gently to his day's work, and then greet whatever arrived at the door, or over the hopping phone. Shock, trauma, sorrow, anger, hostility, aggression, warmth, love and support, it all arrived, along with a constant wave of people. Nana would greet it all. She would smoke only when absorbed in physical work. Washing the floor, or ironing shirts, we would stare fascinated, as she balanced a Park Drive in her mouth and allowed the ash to grow, until it became a perfectly balanced column in her mouth. We all remember her giggling, finding some moments of hilarity to share with each of us to soften our days. We have vivid memories of our mother folded in two, tears rolling down her cheeks, laughing at some story of the day with Nana, having spent a day in a classroom or seeing constituents in Dad's office.

There were many other visitors. John Doran, ex boxer, cook and global traveller, came often. Hearing him open the front door and shout hello, we would start laughing almost before he appeared, knowing he was coming with a funny story and words of kindness. Big Joe Moran would sit for a cup of tea and a bap and ask questions of us children about our days, giving us gentle kind encouragement. Berna, Dad's election agent, exuded strength and resilient certainty. There was an army of strong women around mum and dad during times of campaigning and later, elections. There were also men and women from increasingly influential walks of life who would arrive and often end up staying, experiencing something of the daily intensities of those times.

The fact that every one of the diverse range of people who landed at the door was treated with equal respect by both our parents was a great lesson for us growing up, as reflected in a paragraph in the Nobel acceptance speech:

Difference is the essence of humanity. Difference is an accident of birth, and it should therefore never be the source of hatred or conflict. Therein lies a most fundamental principle of peace: respect for diversity.

Our mother, whose warmth and humanity created an open door and a welcoming space for many – both in our home and in dad's office which she ran from 1979 – showed us the importance of compassion/empathy as everyday practice. She chose to see the lovable and the delight in all situations as far as possible, and has been a role model of warmth, love and resilience for us.

Difficulties encountered in the last few years in politics contributed to our father suffering from many bouts of ill-health. There were many causes of these problems, but it is worth noting here that empathy by itself can be overwhelming and lead to burnout. In order to be sustainable, empathy must be balanced by deep and resilient self-compassion and self-care. We live in times where great divisiveness exists and where the need for action on many global challenges can seem overwhelming. Social media provides scope for abuse and distortion. Self-care and self-compassion are critical. None of us are perfect, we can't fix everything and that's OK.

The latter part of our father's life, as he succumbed to dementia, illustrated the power of empathetic action as multiple small kindnesses. The compassion shown to him by the people of Derry and Donegal, who stopped to talk to him in the street every day, guided him to protect his independence, and received him with gentleness if he was agitated, was a profound gift to our family. This and the care shown to him by the staff in the nursing home where he spent his final days was the best demonstration we could have had of empathy, compassion and love. Over many years, the hordes of strangers who took time to send a message of support, by writing a card or sending a short letter provided strength, light and comfort to our parents through many dark times.

In the fullness of life, we'll all be strong and we'll all be vulnerable. The last years of our father's life underlined to us the importance of a society where kindness, respect and care are central. The work of our parents and the broader community that surrounded them emphasised to us the critical importance of respect for diversity and difference. It taught us the on-going need for listening, and dialogue, to build, maintain and nourish relationships and understanding. When, as it can currently seem, political discourse is limited to competing and divisive versions of righteousness, empathy can help illustrate the blind spots, reimagine the bigger picture and liberate a kinder present. Empathy, tempered with compassionate action, and love for ourselves, each other and the shared kinship of our planetary home, provides a path to help us rethink and reimagine our society so we can better adapt to the myriad challenges we now face.

Empathy. Kindness. The greatest of all wisdom.

Empathy – A True Champion of the West

Marcus Hannick and family

In a small, coastal, North Mayo town in the early 1960s, there was not much for young people to do. This is one of the reasons that on any given day, you may have seen a group of youths playing handball up against a building on a public road, taking it on turns to lookout for any approaching gardaí who would soon put an end to the fun. However, more than once, the assigned watchmen proved ineffective and after several stern warnings from the local town guard, the youths were finally caught, reprimanded, and brought to the local court. Central in this gang of 'hardened criminals' was my father, a sixteen-year-old Seán Hannick.

This incident was the first of many in Seán's life, when he turned an undesirable situation into a positive gain for the greater good of his community. A man who would become hugely influential to Seán throughout his early life, Alfie Reilly was the person who planted the seed. Alfie, a hugely intelligent man, had been studying medicine at the time, though he eventually had to forego this due to his own health issues. Once word got out of the 'handball incident', Alfie put it simply to my father, 'sure why don't you build your own handball alley?' and there began Seán's first mission.

The first hurdle lay in acquiring the funding and from this was born the idea of the now infamous Showbands Marquee. Sean got to work organising some of the biggest names in the Irish showband circuit – such as Joe Dolan, Larry Cunningham, the Dixies and Big Tom to come and perform in a marquee, erected in a field just outside Killala town, and the 'John Mortar Society' was set up to secure its funding. These Easter and summer nights were a huge success within the community and were the beginning of a new lifeline for the town, attracting people from all over Ireland. By 1965, due to the success of these events, the handball alley was built in Killala and by 1967 it became only the third roofed alley in the country at that time. This was only the start of the achievements for both Killala and a young Seán Hannick, echoing his favourite line 'what the mind can conceive, the body can achieve', an ethos that he lived by and instilled in those around him for the rest of his life.

Seán had an ability to sense what was needed in his community and in people. He looked around and saw possibilities, opportunities to help, improve and grow. He knew that understanding people, their needs and their problems, was crucial in making change happen. His goal was bettering the community and to achieve this, developing people and their own individual abilities was key.

My father was born in 1943, the only child of the local butcher, Johnny, and his loving wife Matilda (fondly known as Tilly). He worked in the butcher shop from a very young age, observing how his father showed kindness to the less fortunate of his customers. He was tough, but fair, giving people help when they needed it. Although initially attending boarding school in St Nathy's in Ballaghaderreen, Seán's formal education was cut short at the age of fourteen when Tilly suffered a stroke, and soon after Johnny passed away. Seán became Killala's new butcher boy, learning to manage the business and all that came with it.

In the 1950s, Killala faced huge challenges like many other rural towns in the west of Ireland. Particularly for young people, there were few opportunities or prospects. However, with the arrival of the aforementioned 'marquee era' of the 1960s, things in Killala began to look up. Seán loved how the success of the marquees energised the place and saw what could be achieved with hard work, community spirit and people working together. This was almost a golden era for the town, kickstarting numerous landmark projects spearheaded by Seán. One of the most striking things about all of this was the way in which he conducted his leadership based on the instinctive empathy he had towards others. These projects put Killala on the national and eventually the global map.

One of the first of these was in 1959 when he became involved in the Harbour Committee, which was set up to help local farmers afford the unattainable rising cost of fertiliser by organising bulk orders to be shipped into Killala Bay from Norway at a much lower cost. Then in 1978, Killala Community Centre was founded – a hugely important development in the history of the town. Prompted by a newspaper advertisement he saw for government grants being offered to build commumnity recreational centres, Seán drove to Dublin to put in an application. He then went straight to the Minister for Finance at the time, to ask him for the £240,000 to build it. The minister, impressed with his determination and sheer boldness, gave him £140,000 and left it with Seán to fundraise the rest, which together with the community, he did. To this day Killala Community Centre is a fundamental and essential part of the community.

Seán was also instrumental in eventually opening up Killala to international waters, when the Japanese synthetic fiber plant of Asahi was opened in the town in 1974. Perhaps one of the most significant developments in the town's history. Along with the IDA and The Community Council, he knew the overwhelmingly positive effect this would, and did, have on the area. Seán fought hard to get this opportunity into the town, and it eventually employed 350 people. The arrival of Asahi created what can only be described as a mini 'Celtic Tiger' for the west of Ireland, bringing huge prosperity and development to the area, at a time of huge emigration and recession in the rest of Ireland.

Dad also played a significant role in the establishment of the Ceide Fields Heritage Centre. Local Professor, Seamus Caufield knew that North Mayo lay home to a huge area of historical interest, where a Neolithic site containing the oldest known stone-walled fields in the world (dating back 6,000 years) were located. He also knew that to create what is now an award-winning landmark, he would need to enlist the help of someone who never saw any task as too big to achieve. Seán led the way in raising the significant sum and becoming chairman of the committee, and the Ceide Fields is still one of Ireland's main historical tourist attractions today.

The success of this soon called for Seamus and Seán's leadership again in 1991 in the formation of the Foxford Woollen Mills. During a meeting to brainstorm the project, when the amount of money needed was realised, the attendees were shocked and disheartened. A serene Seán grabbed a cigarette box from someone and on the back of it calmly wrote a breakdown of where they could come up with the money, from grants to fundraising. Soon the entire monetary breakdown was outlined and planned out, right there on a packet of Major.

These are just some of the many, many projects, developments, and opportunities that Seán worked so hard to bring to his community. Some others included the Advanced Factories Scheme, numerous Housing Developments in the town, Chicago Bridge and Iron, *The Year of the French* filmed in Killala and the Fish Co-op. Seán was always wondering what more could be done for people and never thought twice about putting any idea, no matter how big or seemingly unachievable it was, into action. So much so, that the town of Killala soon gained recognition at a European level. In 1978, it was chosen as a case study by professors at the University of Galway together with Penn State University in the US, demonstrating how this small town was the leader in all of Europe for social and community development. I often think about how my father's empathy for the people in his community and desire to make life better for them led to such huge successes.

Seán was a natural leader; his positivity had a profound impact on people and his ability to consistently get the best out of people was remarkable. Be it through persuasion, collective motivation or purely giving an individual a purpose and trusting in that person by giving them responsibility and ownership, Seán's empowering leadership style progressively developed individuals and groups.

The list of achievements stands as testimony to the selflessness of my father as he set about trying to improve the lives of the people of our local region and beyond. He pursued his goals with unquenchable spirit but with great modesty, immense patience, and never-failing grace.

Above all, it was the empathy in everything he did that earned him the many extraordinary tributes that followed his passing. The archive facts, stories, and many examples of the work he carried out so diligently and so discreetly in his trademark fashion, became a son's fascination with the man he knew as his father and would later become an exemplar for life and success.

Managers of Empathy

Paul McGrath

In many ways the Ireland of my youth in the 1960s and 1970s was a very different place and time. Unfortunately, many discriminations which existed then, persist to this day, along with new ones, against any sort of difference be that skin colour, gender, religious beliefs or sexuality. Many people are still targeted or omitted for a variety of reasons and as a result can find life very hard.

Growing up, I always felt different and a bit of an outsider which regularly left me isolated and affected my confidence. I found it difficult to find a place where I felt comfortable. For me, through some very close friendships and the support of a number of key people at the time, I found a place which gave me a home and a place to grow in football.

Football allowed me to be myself and was somewhere I could work hard to develop the base skill I had been given. Over time, I was lucky to make a professional career in a sport I love. This would not have been possible without a variety of support and acts of kindness from some key people along the way that gave me the confidence and opportunity to develop this career. It has also given me great friends.

I played football for my local teams, then for St Patrick's Athletic before I was given the chance to pursue my dream and play professional football in England with Manchester United.

Professional football is often not the most welcoming of environments for people who may not conform to the status quo in the dressing-room. Accordingly, it is vital to have people in your corner who will ensure that your personality and individuality is accepted.

I had a number of physical injuries over the years which limited my ability to train as other players could. I also have had, and continue to have, my own personal challenges off the football pitch. These are well documented and as I have tried to work through a difficult time, I have not always behaved as I should. However, whenever I have needed a helping hand at such times, I am grateful to have found this from a number of close people who understood that I may have needed help in a different way.

I have been very fortunate that Irish football fans have always given me incredible support, both in a football sense and beyond. This continues to this day when I am out and about – the warmth I feel from them always gives me a huge lift. Within football there have been people associated with each of my clubs who have watched out for me.

There are two people in particular who always had the awareness to give me a leg up when I needed it most. Their support was often provided in a subtle way, sometimes never verbalised but I knew that through their action or indeed on occasion their inaction, that their support was rock solid.

The first was one of my managers at Aston Villa, Graham Taylor. Graham was a leading manager in the English game and subsequently went on to manage England. One of his biggest strengths was in his management of his players. Despite his high profile, Graham made time to get to know his players, and to be aware of what was going on in their lives. He had the compassion to make concessions he felt would help that person both on and off a football pitch. I will never forget his kindness.

The second person, which will not surprise most, was my international manager Jack Charlton. I loved playing for my country. Despite winning trophies and awards in England, my greatest pride was in being given the chance to represent Ireland. For most of my international career, I was lucky to be managed by Jack Charlton. Jack may have won the World Cup as a player with his native England but he is rightly loved in Ireland for how he led us all through a very exciting time for Irish football.

From early on, Jack realised that I needed certain support and he reached out and put his big arms around me to protect me from myself and occasionally from the media to allow me the space to recover. His protection never waivered despite me testing his commitment once or twice!

In return for the kindness from both Graham and Jack, I worked hard to repay their faith and it is no coincidence that I played some of the best football of my career under them. Without both these men, I would not have had the opportunity to play as many games or to achieve what I was very lucky to do in the professional game.

When you fall outside of the perceived norm or somebody is giving you a hard time, it is so important that somebody has the awareness to show you some compassion, to try to understand the challenge you are facing and by simply taking that interest, to help to improve your lot.

Sadly, both of these great men have passed away in recent years, but I have learned a lot from them in understanding how and when to show empathy with those who need it. I have tried to follow their example in how I behave towards others and endeavour to pass on the empathy that was shown to me on many occasions.

For many people, life can be harsh and lonely and we all need people to be aware of what others are facing and reach out to them to make their lives a small bit easier.

Mary Elmes

Clodagh Finn

It is difficult to capture the spirit of Mary Elmes in words because it was her actions, rather than what she said, that resonate eight decades after she and her colleagues risked their lives to save an estimated 427 children from deportation to Nazi murder camps during the Second World War.

When a bridge was named in her honour in her native city in Cork in 2019, it struck me that one way to appreciate the magnitude of what she did was to visualise all the people she helped to save standing on it. I imagined them all, standing shoulder to shoulder, across the city's magnificent new pedestrian bridge when it opened on a day in late September. Not just the people themselves, but their children and their children's children. They would have crossed the River Lee several times over.

'Whoever saves a life saves the world entire,' as the famous Talmud teaching goes.

Mary Elmes' bravery, humanity and empathy live on in them and, most poignantly, her spirit continues to ripple down through the generations in the most unexpected ways.

To give one particularly moving example, one mother's last words – spoken out the window of a train en route to Auschwitz death camp – found their way to a child saved by Mary Elmes seventy-five years later because they were valued and put in an archive.

On 4 September 1942, the train carrying Polish woman Zirl Berger (31) stopped briefly at Montauban, near Toulouse in France. A colleague of Mary's, Nora Cornelissen, was standing on the platform with others, hoping to provide some comfort to those within. In that snatched moment, Zirl Berger managed to get a message to her daughter. 'Send her my most affectionate thoughts and a thousand kisses,' she said.

Days earlier, Mary Elmes had spirited away that little girl to a place of safety, La Villa St-Christophe, one of the children's homes she initially set up to offer respite from the harsh conditions at Rivesaltes holding camp in south-west France, but which became vital safe houses as deportations began.

Charlotte Berger-Greneche stayed at the Villa for a short time before spending her childhood in other similar homes. She has happy memories of those places, but none at all of her mother, bar a faint memory of being dressed by her in Rivesaltes camp. All her life, she had neither photo nor memento of the woman who brought her into the world in 1937.

Her mother's words, however, were faithfully recorded by Mary's colleague Nora Cornelissen and later filed away in the archive of the American Friends Service Committee (the AFSC or American Quakers), a vast repository that shines a light on the work Mary Elmes was so reluctant to speak of in later life.

By sheer chance, I came across them months after interviewing Charlotte Berger-Greneche in 2017 while researching a biography of Mary Elmes. A miraculous needle in a very dark haystack. I sent her mother's message to her on 6 May 2017. This was the message that came back: 'It is the most moving message I've had. A thousand thank-yous.'

It is hard to estimate exactly how many people Mary and her colleagues saved. From August to October 1942, some 2,289 Jewish adults and 174 children, some as young as two, were herded onto cattle wagons and taken from Rivesaltes holding camp to Drancy in Paris and then on to the gas chambers of Auschwitz in Poland.

Those numbers would be even higher had it not been for the work of Mary's organisation, the AFSC, the Red Cross and a French charity, OSE (Oeuvre de Secours aux Enfants). According to one estimate, some 427 children were saved from deportation from Rivesaltes camp. We know that Mary Elmes hid a family in her own flat in Perpignan too, and she also arranged documents and visas for hundreds of others.

Of those deported from the camp Mary knew so well, fewer than 100 survived.

The story of the Second World War is one of repugnant brutality and state-sponsored persecution and murder. The Holocaust claimed the lives of more than six million Jewish people and as many others who were murdered on political, ideological or racial grounds. Alongside that horror, though, are many often-untold stories of the people who showed extraordinary courage to help others, risking their own lives to do so.

We might know nothing of Mary Elmes had it not been for Professor Ronald Friend who nominated her for Israel's highest honour, Righteous Among the Nations, having found out that she was the one who saved him and his brother Michael 'from certain death', as he puts it.

A passage in the diary of Lois Gunden, who ran the children's home La Villa Saint-Christophe with Mary, offers a glimpse into how these exceptional women tried to spare children the trauma of war, not to mention save their lives. In 1942, Lois estimated that every two or three weeks, Mary brought between three and seven children to the home. On 11 August, for instance, she recorded the arrival of seven children:

> While we were eating supper Miss Elmes brought seven Jewish

> children – some of whom can't speak French; Mussoles cooked some extra macaroni; *quelle comédie pour les laver en lavabo!* [what theatrics when we went to wash them in the washbasin]. *Les garçons ne voulaient pas enlever leurs culottes* [The boys didn't want to take off their underpants]; finally found bed spare for everyone; 43 in house at present …

The theatrics with the boys' underpants was a chilling reminder of how parents had warned their circumcised sons not to undress to hide the fact that they were Jewish.

Both women knew their work was putting them in immediate and real danger. A few months after the deportations were complete, Mary Elmes was arrested by the German security police and accused of a series of hostile acts against the Reich. She spent six months in a Gestapo prison, but she made little of that in later life, saying: 'Well, we all experienced inconveniences in those days, didn't we?'

That was typical of her. She refused all accolades in her lifetime and spoke little of her work during the Second World War or in the Spanish Civil War in the years before it. She told her children, Caroline and Patrick Danjou, snippets as they grew up in Perpignan where she lived all her life, having married Frenchman Roger Danjou in 1946.

Author Rosemary Bailey was the first person to write about her in English in her book *Love and War in the Pyrenees* in 2008. Since then, thanks to researchers Bernard and Janet Wilson, a Quaker couple with a deep interest in Mary Elmes and her work, the archive of the AFSC has been more widely read.

The risks Mary Elmes took during the Second World War often capture the headlines, but it was in an earlier conflict, the Spanish Civil War, that she gained a reputation as a shrewd and able administrator who was clear-headed and unsentimental in war. She volunteered as an aid worker in Spain in 1937, moving eastwards – from Almería to Murcia, Alicante and Polop – as the fascist army advanced, setting up and running children's hospitals as she went.

She had excelled in modern languages (Spanish and French) in Trinity College, Dublin, an experience that instilled in her a lasting love of Spain. Her exceptional grades won her a scholarship to the London School of Economics and later Geneva. When the Spanish Civil War broke out in 1936, she felt compelled to help the Spanish people.

She said, at one point, she went there because she wanted to know the Spanish people better. She said she admired their enthusiasm and unquenchable spirit.

We might say the same of her. More than that, what is striking is how that spirit lives on. In 2019, Charlotte Berger-Greneche, the little girl Mary saved in 1942, travelled to Cork to attend the opening of the Mary Elmes bridge. She was joined by Georges Koltein who, along with his brother Jacques, also found sanctuary in one of Mary's children's homes. Both of them visited Mary Elmes' former school, Ashton in Cork city, where Charlotte told the assembled 520 pupils not to forget the past.

'We have to take the lessons of the past because things can always happen again. We have to be very careful,' she said. I will never forget the silence in the auditorium as the softly spoken then eighty-year-old spoke, nor the thunderous standing ovation that followed.

It was, I think, the essence of how human empathy can be passed on like a baton, from Mary Elmes to Charlotte Berger-Greneche and from Charlotte to the next generation. May it ripple on.

Finding Empathy in a World gone Mad

Eamonn Fitzgerald

Most mornings, on my walk to work, I pass by my elderly neighbour, a retired civil servant, sitting in his porch reading a newspaper. Sometimes I would see him take a small notebook out of his jacket pocket and write something in it. He would then put the notebook back in his pocket and continue to read his paper. Most evenings, walking home from work, when the weather was fine, I would see him again out tending to his garden. Sometimes I would stop for a socially distant neighbourly chat.

One day, as curiosity got the better of me, I asked him if he was keeping a diary. He beckoned me into his garden, took out his battered notebook, and thumbed through it to me today's entry. It was simply today's date and the number 1763. Seeing the confused look on my face, he explained that every morning he would look for the amount of people that had died as a result of the pandemic and record the total in his notebook. He told me he would take some time to sit for a while and think about all the people that were affected by these deaths. He would then say a prayer for them to help 'their souls into eternity'.

Since the pandemic had started, he felt the world was tinged with sadness and it needed something positive to help it. As he was isolating, he said the best he could do for these people was to say a prayer for them and their families. He said he wasn't going to let this pandemic change the person he was. He genuinely felt upset by what was going on around him and felt he wanted to do something to help, and all he could was offer his thoughts and prayers. It was his way of coping.

This got me thinking about how I was coping during the pandemic. I work as a grocery manager. Since the pandemic started, we have become busier than we ever have been historically. I was never locked down. We ended up working harder than we ever did before with less staff. We had double digit growth, and hundreds more pallets of stock were coming in the back door every week and all of the stock had to be put on shelves and sold. Everyone remembers the empty shelves at the start of the pandemic, the queuing to get into the shops, and the general sense of panic people had. As the workload increased, my management team and my staff (so-called essential workers) became more stressed and short-tempered. We were trying to balance an increased workload, with social distancing, angry customers, and sick calls. With the increased absenteeism, I was called into work on my days off. As time went by, I was becoming more overwhelmed at work and I was tired all the time. Work fatigue had set in. I was no longer happy doing my job.

Customers who initially 'clapped for the essential workers' were now incredibly abusive to the staff as they tried to cope with the increased workloads. Nobody wanted to work in 'customer service' as they took quite an amount of abuse from customers. I dreaded being called to Customer Service as is usually meant dealing with an angry customer. The retail environment had become (and still is) quite a toxic place to work in. When the mask mandate came in, it increased the stress levels even more as some customers refused to wear masks and maintain the required social distancing. Staff turn-over increased. The managers were all bickering and fighting each other. Morale was at an all-time low. I personally was finding it hard to relate to people any more, even to 'understand where they were coming from'. I knew everyone was stressed, but I didn't react to it as my own stress levels were beginning to overwhelm me. I hated going into work, and I had a short temper all the time. My work life began to affect my home life, as I was the only member of the family not isolating. I was coming home stressed and this would be passed on to the family.

My conversations with my elderly neighbour and the arguments at home made me realise I wasn't coping very well, I didn't even recognise that my staff weren't coping very well, and worse of all, I didn't recognise that my family was under pressure too. In fact, I'd started not to care about anyone as I was trying to block out all the uncomfortable emotions around me. I was experiencing what I now understand to be 'empathy overload' or 'empathy distress'. My coping mechanism was simply to block out all the negativity and respond to every situation with anger. I needed to take back some control of my life. I needed to help myself before I could help others. I needed to get my empathy back.

As a manager of a large team, I always prided myself in knowing what was going on in everyone's mind. For example, I knew who was going to do exams, so needed time off. I knew who didn't get on with whom, so I could manage the roster to have a smooth work day for everybody. I fixed problems before they started. I had the right people in the right place at the right time. I understood people had issues at home and would accommodate them with time off. I carefully listened, coached and praised every staff member, enforcing the concept of 'we're all in this together, and we're as strong as the weakest link'. I didn't let the team down and they didn't let me down either. I did my best to keep a smooth productive workplace where people wanted to work and get on. Then the pandemic struck.

I over time became completely overwhelmed and stressed and changed my management style to a more draconian style. I stopped being the empathetic 'hard-nose but fair' manager and just became an angry manager. I was angry all the time and this reflected in the staff performance, which made me angrier and more stressed. I had to change or I knew I would burn-out.

Six months into the pandemic, I started my journey to become the manager I was before everything changed. I knew the pandemic had changed me. I knew I was 'good with people' and I'd forgotten how I used to do it. I realised I had lost my important management skill; my ability to have empathy to others. Empathy is having a capacity to understand or feel what another person is experiencing from within their frame of reference. In a nutshell, it is an ability to put you in another person's shoes and understanding or feeling what they must be feeling. Sometimes you can be overloaded by other people, but you can learn strategies to help.

I started by thinking about how I used to interact with staff and how I was interacting with them now:

• I was good at listening to what staff would say to me. I always asked open-ended questions. As I was so stressed, I hadn't time to listen to anyone, and problems I would normally quite easily solve myself, I would simply refer the staff to the HR department.

• Staff would often tell me non-work related personal problems. I would never judge them and I would do my best to help them. Again, as I had enough of my own problems, and I didn't want to hear any of their problems.

• I would be able to pick up what others were feeling and I would often think about what they were feeling in the hope I could do something to help them a little bit. Now I didn't want to talk to anyone. I didn't want to take on anyone else's problems.

• Regularly staff came to me to ask for advice in non-work related matters. I noticed that recently nobody was actually talking to me about anything that wasn't related to work. People were actually avoiding me and I was quite happy they were.

• I realised that this pandemic was overwhelming me, and I was letting it. As a result, I was projecting my stress levels on the staff. Productivity and morale plummeted,

• At one time, I knew I actually cared about the staff. I had wanted each one of them to develop to the best of their ability, to take pride in the work they do, and I would regularly give good praise and positive feedback. Right now, I didn't care about anyone as long as the work was done. I found myself telling people over and over to just 'get it done'.

• I had not so rigid boundaries with the staff – I encouraged them to reach out if they needed me. Now I didn't want to interact with them and didn't even go into the canteen any more. On my breaks, I went out to the car park and sat there. Once my shift was over, I would clock out immediately and go home.

• I found making social connections at work had become more difficult. Especially with the new staff who stayed away from me, as they perceived me to be a very angry manager. They were afraid of me and I didn't care.

In essence, I was no longer calm at work. I had lost my ability to have some form of emotional regulation (I used to pride myself in my ability to experience the pressures and stress of working in a fast-paced retail environment without becoming in any way overwhelmed). This needed to change.

Looking at the above list, I realised I needed to re-connect with my management and staff teams. From a business point of view, if I looked after my internal customers first (staff and management), then we could look after the external customers better. I had to calm down again. I had to become de-stressed and manage the feelings of being overwhelmed. So I started by asking people questions and listening to the answers. Some of the questions I asked included:

• Are you ok? This was met initially by surprise, but when I explained how I was stressed but was trying to cope with it, they were willing to tell me how stressed they were. Once they realised I was trying to go back to the calm state I used to be in, they recognised this and started to calm down too.

• What can we do to make the job easier? Once the staff understood I was genuinely trying to help them to get through the phenomenal amount of work we had to do every day, they offered some positive feedback. We changed some work practices to make the work easier. Staff felt empowered as they got away from the idea of 'that's how we always did it' to finding a better way of doing things.

• How are you feeling/coping? The results varied from not so good, to actually not so bad. The staff who were coping the best gave me advice which I could share with the staff that were having a hard time.

• We actually are all in this together. I would tell everyone to work together, help each other, and we'd get through this. We'd got this far and there was no reason why we wouldn't see this to the end.

• How are your family coping? Some staff would tell me about members of their family being ill, and I try to remember and ask them about their family members a few days later. If the needed time off, I would try my best to accommodate them. Even if I couldn't help them with time off, the fact I'd asked meant a lot.

• What can you do to help the guy coming into this area to work after you go home? In retail, the job is never ending. There is always another shelf to pack. This was important that the staff would leave the area like they found it or in a better condition. They began to realise the importance of everyone helping everyone.

Most of the questions asked were to try to re-connect with the team, to try to build a sense of team spirit so we would help each other get through this. The more as a manager that I interacted and connected with the staff, the more the moral and productivity seemed to improve. The old adage of 'leading by example' was true. If I was calm, then everyone was calm. If I worked hard, everyone worked hard.

People commented that it had been a while since they saw me taking off my jacket and rolling up my sleeves to 'get stuck in'. I realised that my increased levels of empathy were important as it connected the staff together into a team in the sense that no one felt left out, and there was a sense that we were all in this together, rowing the boat in the same direction. As my personal levels of distress and stress decreased, it decreased in the team around me. People started to talk to me again. Problems were solved before they became an issue, and work became a better place again.

I was able to ask the staff, once they realised I was trying to deal with this difficult time too, what they wanted in an effective manager or what they wanted to see in the management team. I'd forgotten what was important to the staff and I made another list of some of their replies:

• A good manager recognised that staff members are people and not numbers. People have feelings and these need to be recognised.

• The manager is always calm under pressure and is willing to listen to suggestions to problems as they arise.

• The manager is ethical in his behaviour. They always strive to be a positive influence to everyone else.

• They are kind and have a positive set of morals.

• The manager always considers the needs of others along with the needs of the business.

• A good manager will use professional language at all times, not forgetting the please and thank-you good manners.

• A good manager will take risks for the team – for example going against a head office direction if it is seen to be offensive to the staff.

• A good manager is seen to have a strong desire to make a positive difference and to positively develop the staff.

• A good manager is seen to be consistent, professional, and above all fair.

Initially, it was hard for me to calm down, to return to the empathetic management style I had practised for nearly thirty years. I had to begin to listen to my team again, to gently encourage and develop them. I asked many positive open-ended questions and implemented the positive feedback. I was beginning to feel less stressed by my environment. I had taken some control back. My work life has improved. Consequently, my home life has improved too. The journey back has been difficult, but I'm glad I took it.

I still pass my elderly neighbour every day, and I've told him about how my personal and work life has improved as a result of the decision I made to return to my old empathic management style. He's happy that something positive came out of our conversations. He's still writing in his notebook and at the time of writing the number is now 5,000. We both hope it won't increase much further.

I'm less stressed and as a result less tired. I have a better work life-balance. I feel I can get through the rest of this pandemic without being overwhelmed, and in fact I now believe I will come out of it a better person than I was when this started. I believe too that my team will come out of it in a better position too, more resilient and united in their efforts – all because of a conversation with a neighbour who had empathy for people all his life and who wouldn't let the pandemic change who he is as a person.

Ciorcal Iomlán

Kathy Hyland

Empathy. A small word, with huge relevance. As I reflect on my life and career to date with the theme of empathy as a backdrop, I struggle to weave and loop the enormity of its significance and impact.

To me empathy and compassion feel intrinsically interlinked. The word compassion originated in the 1300s, with the Latin *compati* translating to 'to suffer with'.

To accompany someone in their suffering moves compassion beyond sympathy, transmuted into the deeper presence of empathy.

A privilege to have experienced in the capacity that I have, and now find myself working in a field where empathy is not only important, it is essential. Awareness of the impact that empathy has had on my life has enriched, inspired and influenced me in ways that are hard to quantify.

Losing a loved one is undoubtedly one of life's most difficult experiences. A loss that becomes a part of us, which we must then find a way to carry alongside with us, in our newly restructured world. Reminders of the loss are everywhere to be found in this new landscape, and empathy experienced on this path helps us to navigate this new territory.

Having experienced the death of my father at a young age, I am reminded of the powerful experiences of empathy that shaped my path, healed my heart and subsequently served as a powerful catalyst to train in the field of Art Therapy.

Attempting to navigate the harsh new landscape of childhood grief, when accompanied by empathy and compassion allows for healing, resilience, acceptance and readjustment. A reminder that although in the depths of turbulent times, there is still good to be found in the world.

I'm not sure if I was aware at the time that what I was experiencing was 'empathy', but I was aware of the effect it had on my life.

This kindness allowed colour and light to return to my world, and its impact has stayed with me as a transformative and powerful influence.

Suffering is a universal experience for us all here in this lifetime, and empathy a universal language.

Art too functions as a language, often revealing our inner worlds and providing us with an alternative language to articulate our life experiences.

During my time spent in Cape Town, South Africa, as a newly qualified Art Therapist, evidence of this was clear. While working with children in the township of Nyanga, and in the oncology and burns unit in The Red Cross Children's Hospital, the language of empathy was central to the therapeutic process.

Empathy became a meeting ground when our native tongues differed, a means of connection, communication and care. Although culturally (and figuratively) miles apart, Art Therapy and empathy transcended barriers, and combined was something understood when words failed.

Working in Palliative care as an Art Therapist is both challenging yet incredibly rewarding. Harrowing at times, yet tinged with some of the most profound and significant moments of love, compassion and empathy. Raw vulnerable emotions simmer through the halls here, as loved one's hearts break on a daily basis.

Oftentimes it feels like empathy and compassion are the

cogs that allow some semblance of normalcy during these difficult days.

When approaching end of life, words alone can often fall short when trying to express the depth and complexity of what is being experienced. Art Therapy is a special and unique way of working that allows space for these feelings and emotions to be expressed through a combination of words and creativity.

Its essence is creative meaningful engagement that provides a gentle yet powerful form of emotional and psychological support. The importance of empathy while supporting patients and family members is paramount to holistic palliative care.

It assists with feeling seen, heard and understood during some of the most difficult times in our lives. When working with children who have experienced trauma and loss, I feel in a profound position of privilege to be able to support them in this way. Being a witness to this pain is a reminder that we are not alone. A reminder of our shared humanity.

Empathy often requires a shift in perspective, to 'tune into' and be sensitive and fully present to the inner world and emotional reality of others, for it is here where our pain and struggle is kept. We can all practise and cultivate empathy in various ways and roles in our lives.

> It is most encouraging to know that this subtle, elusive quality of utmost importance, is not something 'one is born with', but can be learned, and learned most rapidly in an empathic climate.
>
> Carl Rogers, *Empathic: An Unappreciated Way of Being*

Kindness and empathy shown is never forgotten, and its effects and influence are far reaching. Deep empathy is knowledge that we are not all that different and provides an opportunity to sustain each other through the complexities that life continually offers.

Luck

Louis de Paor

Sa *subway* fé bhun
Madison Square Garden
táim im aonar ar deireadh,

dríodar na hoíche aréir
ag suathadh mo chuid fola
is mo chroí á ghreadadh féin:

dornálaí meata
ná cloífeadh mála páipéir.

Díreach is an glór miotail
ag fógairt go bhfuil an traein
ar tí imeachta

réabann fear gorm
tríd an doras
taobh thiar dom

ropann tríd an slua
is amach ceann eile
an chairr.

Tá póilíní anois
ar gach taobh dínn

gunnaí amuigh
is iad ag gabháil
tríd an gcarráiste

chomh ciúin
leis an té atá uathu.

Ar éigin más fiú
le héinne
de na paisinéirí

bacaint
leis an dráma
leadránach marfach

atá feicthe acu
rómhinic cheana
ach tá mo shúile ar cipíní

is mo chroí
á léasadh féin
gan tlás.

Tá dán beag
le Langston Hughes
os cionn an dorais

is mé ar mo dhícheall
ag iarraidh é a léamh
chun mo chladhaire boilg
a chur chun suaimhnis:

Sometimes a crumb falls
From the tables of joy …

Anois nó riamh,
arsa mise liom fhéin:

léigh leat
go bhfeicfidh tú

an bhfuil freagra ar bith
ar an gceist a chuireann

na neamhléitheoirí
neamhfhilíochta ort:

in ainm Dé,
nó cad sa foc
is fiú dán

i ngleann seo
gan trócaire
na ndeor?

Léigh leat, mar adúirt
an file Polainneach,
chomh mall

is dá mbeadh biachlár
á scagadh agat
in óstán galánta:

Sometimes a crumb falls
From the tables of joy
Sometimes a bone
Is flung.

Dúntar na doirse
is bogann an capall iarainn
le gíoscán srathair
sa tollán geimhreata
idir dhá dhoircheacht:

Uaireanta
Titeann blúire aráin
De bhord an áthais
Uaireanta caitear cnámh.

Ar dhaoine áirithe
Bronntar grá
Ar dhaoine eile
Neamh amháin.

No Idea what will Happen Next

Tiernan Henry

Whitesnake played Dublin's SFX hall in February 1984. At the back of the room, that night, was an nineteen-year-old from Dundalk. Six weeks earlier, in the first week of January, she had major surgery in the Richmond, and a couple of months earlier – just before her birthday – she had emergency surgery in Dundalk to stop the bleed from a ruptured ulcer. The bleed was stopped, but the presence, extent and scope of an extensive leiomyosarcoma was revealed, which had her in the Richmond right after New Year. Her surgeon and his team removed the tumours, her pancreas and most of her stomach. In recovery, she was asked if she'd like to meet Bono (who was visiting Luke Kelly). She declined, asking, instead to meet Dave Coverdale.

She was discharged at the end of January, with a short, terse one-page letter from her surgeon that ended simply, we have no idea what will happen next.

For Anne – that nineteen-year-old – going to the SFX was what had to happen next. Pumped full of drugs and terrified her stitches would burst, she wasn't going to miss this gig. And, she was showing that she read the discharge letter as an invitation to live. Breath was what she was craving. More breath. The thing she needed to keep staying alive. And she lived. This funny, smart and gorgeous young woman navigated very complicated waters through her twenties – no idea what will happen next extended to no help in managing a diet with pretty much no stomach, though, as she did point out, the alcohol, cigarettes and dancing covered a lot of ground.

No idea what will happen next included turbulence and loss, then a move to Galway and, fifteen years after we first met as teens, marrying me (fifteen-year-old Anne told one of her sisters that she'd met a boy – sixteen-year-old me – who liked Bob Dylan, but he liked Neil Young too, so he was okay).

Anne Kenny joined COPE Galway in 1997, as a relief worker (the place was coming down with Anns and Annes, so she was – one name – Annekenny). Within the year, she was off to the homeless service, where she worked with families and then began outreach work supporting families experiencing homelessness. This led to a role focused on working with families to sustain tenancies. In 2009, she took on the role of manager of Senior Support Services, where she remained for the next ten years. This summary doesn't even get under the skin of what she learned and what she brought to COPE. In many ways, they were a perfect fit for each other; the focus in COPE is always on supporting the client and advocating for the client's rights. Empathy is there in the foundation of COPE, and Anne's inherently empathic approach blossomed. She was always curious and interested in people, and her lived experience gave her a perspective that found her most comfortable sitting beside people listening to them. She listened easily, reading the room better than anyone I knew – she could make tea and continue to listen and talk, or she could sit and give her full attention to someone, and people just felt relaxed in her company.

She sat beside people, she worked beside them, they did things together and the conversation became part of the normal, and part of work and life. She remembered things people said, she saw their importance and she acknowledged this in different ways. In management, she retained this stance and worked hard to include clients and staff in decision-making and in resolving problems. This inclusive approach made sense to her and seemed entirely logical; she saw this not just as a means of capacity building with clients and staff, but just the right thing.

This empathy based approach emerged for her, almost fully formed, in COPE, because this is how she saw the world. This is how she lived and this is how she interacted with people. In COPE, she found a place where the community work approach matched her approach. Research shows that social workers with previous experiences found an empathy-based approach easier to adopt in practice. Anne found this perfectly natural: she would listen to people and process what they said, she'd support them, help them, and she wasn't afraid to ask difficult questions, because she'd already asked herself similar questions. For her, empathy was the starting point that underpinned practice.

In her twenties and thirties, she had a few short stays in hospitals in Dublin and Galway. She said that, especially in her early twenties, she'd have to constantly retell her story to disbelieving medics and she often said that she wasn't really being listened to – she often felt that she was seen just as a carrier of pain, or illness. She had to learn to push back against this and to get doctors and consultants to engage with her, and not just her diagnosis. This imbalance of power, and the heedlessness stuck with her. Her empathy was inherent, but it was underpinned by experience of being disempowered and of being disbelieved about her lived experience.

The seventeen-year-old Anne had no interest in school and just wanted away. After her surgeries, she went full tilt at life. She wasn't careless or reckless, but she felt she'd been given room to breathe and room to live. No idea what will happen next, let her cut loose and push the sky back.

It also led her to an Open University degree in Social

Science that took her to an MSc in Family Support Studies, working with Pat Dolan. She started a PhD but after a year she returned to COPE; she loved the research, but she missed the hurly burly of work in COPE much more, and back she went. What the University of Galway gave her was a research and academic framework for what she had been doing for years, it gave her a lexicon, and a vocabulary for what she had learned herself, and ways to reflect on her practice. She built clouds of support – she found like minds in COPE, in the University of Galway, in city council, everywhere. And she found the people she needed who could help a client or colleague, and she worked hard to win them over or wring support from them.

No idea what will happen next brought Anne to COPE, and she developed deep and strong friendships across the organisation, in the University of Galway and pretty much everywhere she spent time. In Ann Patchett's words, Anne could always see people at their best and most complete selves. Empathy is the ability to understand and share others' feelings; it's about awareness, intuition, reflective thought and emotional intelligence. Anne was all of those, and more.

No idea what will happen next was also a diagnosis that her cancer had returned in 2015. Chemotherapy and surgery followed. And she was still working the room. Nurses, doctors and catering staff sat and talked to her and she listened to their stories, and her hospital rooms rang with laughter.

In January 2020, Anne died. Her impact on so many people was profound and that will be carried forward. Paraphrasing Auden:

> The current of her feeling had failed;
> she has become her admirers.

Mendelson, E. (Ed) 1991. W.H. Auden: *Collected Poems*. Random House, NY.

Epilogue: Reflections on Learning Empathy

Mark Brennan and Pat Dolan

Ar scáth a chéile a mhaireann na daoine.

(Under the shadow of each other, people survive)

Proverb

This final essay brings us to the end of this book … but not the end of this journey to ensure a movement for empathy in Ireland. The essays and poems presented here are not feel-good stories deigned to simply excite the reader. They are a reminder to all of us of how important, and central, empathy is to our lives and well-being. Empathy has not just shaped our lives – it has also helped create stronger families and ultimately enhanced communities. We hope that sharing the important life experiences presented here, launches a movement and revolution for the development of empathy in Ireland and beyond. Much more important, this is a movement and revolution led by you, in your everyday actions and by the people you inspire.

In this the final essay, we want to do three things:

First, we want to show how empathy is real and critically important to our society. This book was not an academic exercise or a book full of optimistic essays. We work as academics who have researched empathy for over a decade, and put it into practice through programmes and policy. We want to show you the real, tangible and measurable impact that empathy has on individuals and communities. Empathy IS important. Not just in a casual sense, but in a deeply personal and proven way that makes individual lives and communities infinitely healthier. Your empathetic actions, no matter how big or small, have massive impacts that reverberate long, long after you act.

Second, for us, this book served its purpose. It made us even more aware of how acts of empathy and compassion affect our everyday lives. We hope you have found the same. The stories included here vividly opened our eyes to the countless ways in which empathy shapes all of us. And while we have studied empathy for years, this book taught us more than we thought we ever knew. We want to share how the compilation of this book has affected us.

Third, at the end of an inspirational book like this, all of us are left with the questions 'What now?' 'What can I do?' or 'How do I make empathy a reality for myself and others?' We will suggest some ways in which you can use and show empathy in your life and make it part of the lives of others. All are based in proven research and practice experiences. Just remember, no act of empathy is too big or too small. What is vital is that you act with empathy as often as you can … and hopefully more. We are not hoping you spread empathy, we as an Irish society are counting on it. We need you!

WHY EMPATHY?

It takes more courage to dig deep in the dark corners of your own soul and the back alleys of your society than it does for a soldier to fight on the battlefield.

WILLIAM BUTLER YEATS

The expression and receiving of empathy is perhaps the central and most important factor in all aspects of individual and societal development. It is the basis for self-worth, healthy families, productive friendships and strong communities. All significantly affect our own well-being. Simply, empathy is the foundation of functioning societies, our personal development and the gifts we chose to contribute to the world most directly.

Empathy has been described as a response to the emotional state or condition of others and the self. It involves understanding and accepting what the other person is feeling or would be expected to feel. But most simply, it is the capacity to care for another by emotionally 'walking in their shoes'. It is also seen as a key social skill as it allows us to anticipate, understand and experience others' point of view. Empathy is widely understood as encompassing both cognitive ability (the ability to understand the emotions of another) and affective traits (the ability to experience the emotions of another person).

LOST EMPATHY, LOST HUMANITY

Globally, we know that empathy values, social concern and civic engagement are declining across generations because of the increasing individualisation of society over recent decades. Given the importance of empathy and related pro-social values to social cohesion and democracy, it can be argued that it is very important that the value of empathy and care towards others are not lost or left unnurtured. Empathy is at the core of the real lives lived, and crafts embraced, by the writers in this book and provides a promise of healthier communities and societies.

THE PROMISE OF EMPATHY AS 'THE SECRET SAUCE'

Despite perceived declines in empathy and empathetic action, conversely, we are aware that empathy persists everywhere. We also know that it benefits all of us in different ways every day of our lives from global to individual levels. Empathy and reciprocal support with fellow human beings, provides the foundation upon which positive social understanding and care are built.

Empathy is the bread and butter of our relationships and enables us all to thrive across all parts of our existence. In terms of its social benefits, research evidence affirms that the development of empathy is essential to healthy social and emotional functioning and is related to positive social, psychological and personal development, which in turn contributes to the enrichment of civic society.

Where levels of empathy are compromised, studies have found an increased propensity to engage in anti-social behaviour, such as bullying, aggression and violence. Given the importance of empathy to social cohesion and integration, and the emerging evidence regarding the successful teaching of empathy in other countries, it can be argued it is of vital importance that values of empathy and care towards others are given both attention in the formal and informal education systems and promoted across all generations and civic society.

At the individual level, empathy is critical to shaping our responses and perspective toward life, and in shaping our passions, professions, and the craft of where we choose to place our attentions. Importantly we now know that we have a pre-disposition to be empathetic and compassionate, and that we can learn empathy.

The provision and expression of empathy has been the saving point for many of us as individuals. Be this at the family, friends, community or other levels, our lives would have been far different, and likely far sadder, without the empathy of others. These social and psychological impacts of empathy are increasingly documented and transcend not only personal psychological development, but also critical areas such as educational attainment, positive social behaviour, improved mental health, decreased loneliness, and the care provided to those in need.

The expression of empathy has been at the core of our common work. Whether it be in theatre/film, music, teaching, culinary arts, literature, research, comedy, art and other outlets, empathy has been the mechanism for us connecting to the wider world, sharing our own joys and sorrows, providing bonds and comfort, and conveying a common human connectedness. It is the social currency of our lives. It is also the mechanism for applied humanity enabling social support, kindness, awareness raising and the advocacy fight for human rights [and justice]. Utilising the platform our various crafts provide to us, through our work, we can act on behalf of others, meet their needs, enable positive change and present alternatives for a better world to a wider audience. This is not just to the benefit of others, but is in all our interests. Through our work, we see empathy exhibited by chefs feeding people, writers, musicians, teachers and actors entertaining and telling the story of others, artists interpreting a world through paint and sculpture, and comedians offering insight and commentary on the routine and nuanced aspects of our shared humanity.

HOW THIS BOOK SHAPED US

Your battles inspired me – not the obvious material battles but those that were fought and won behind your forehead.

JAMES JOYCE

We witnessed a strange (or maybe not so strange) process in working on this book. First, we approached people we've known and others we've read about, people who at least on the surface appeared to have been deeply impacted by empathy. For those who accepted our offer to be part of the book, we met briefly with everyone. After each single meeting, we were left dumbstruck, star struck, humbled and in awe.

Throughout these talks, the enormity of empathy left us speechless. These people, from all walks of life, had seen everything, experienced everything and were razor sharp focused on the right truth. The real truth of empathy. Their lives, craft and the path that they had chosen, were intertwined with empathy. It was their most powerful weapon to make the world [and themselves] better.

We continuously left each meeting as a fan. Big fans. The kind of fans that needed to investigate everything the people ever did. Every interview, podcast, YouTube video and interview was devoured. We couldn't read enough about them and searched the internet for more insight into their personalities, lives, adventures and actions. Our awe wasn't based in their status, awards or any such things. We joyfully reverted to being like two fifteen-year-olds trying to know everything about our favourite rock stars. It was based in their complete humility and non-negotiable dedication to empathy as the true path forward to make the world better. We remain in wonder of their massive, unparalleled, impact on the human condition.

In all essays, we were allowed to step into the lived lives of others for a moment. You've no doubt experienced such feelings as you read this book. Regardless of our favourites, the process was the same for each one. We became 'them' for a moment, and the world opened up to us. We lived many lives through this book, and we will never … ever … be the same. The world now exists in a nearly inconceivable spectrum of identities and lived lives. All secure (even if not in their own minds) of being on the true path to advancing the human condition, by the decisive action of empathy and active understanding of each other. They all have changed the world in many undervalued ways.

Where do we go from here?

The ordinary acts we practise every day at home are of more importance to the soul than their simplicity might suggest.

Thomas Moore

All of us wonder what we can do to make life better for ourselves and others in a world that seems so complex, challenging and at times difficult. The essays in this book and our years of research and programmes show a clear trend: your empathetic actions, no matter how big or small, have massive impacts. We rarely know how these affect people and communities, but they reverberate long, long after we act.

You've read many examples of how empathy is given, received and how it can be viewed and acted upon. For now, we offer a recipe for empathy that comprises the follow simple steps:

Understanding it
Practising it
Thinking about barriers and overcoming them
Keep doing it!

This book gave many examples for all of these. Use these as a guide as you embrace the art and craft of giving and receiving empathy. You'll do amazing things. The most important thing is that you keep trying!

Final ... or not so final words!

Don't look for meaning in the words. Listen to the silences.

Samuel Beckett

This book is a start in what we hope is a long-term revaluing, sharing and understanding of the central aspect of empathy that cuts across all our lives. Despite all our many perceived differences and lived experiences, we are identical in our need for empathy, social support and a common connection. This is how we survive, overcome adversity, trauma and loss, and ultimately how we can thrive.

For many of us, we have witnessed first-hand the forever powerful impact of empathy in the direst of situations and the recovery from them. Be it in response to childhood trauma and loss, or comprehending 9/11, war, poverty, or the Covid-19 pandemic, empathy has seen us through and empowered us to be positive, constructive, global citizens. Much more important, we look back to history. Faced with war, disease, disaster, terrorism and other threats, those that are remembered for making a difference are those who showed compassion, kindness and empathy to fellow human beings in their greatest hours of need. At Christmas 1914, it even temporarily stopped a World War for a time. Today, compassion, empathy and kindness are at the core of our capacity to respond and recover from any current crisis and can be our anchor and inoculation as we face inevitable future challenges.

We came to this book with simple goals. The research literature, practice knowledge from our crafts and our lived experiences speak volumes about the importance of empathy. We also recognise and remain keenly aware of the important role that empathy played in our own lives. As such, we seek to ensure that empathy education is provided at all levels and for everyone, through schools, community organisations, adult education settings, and other settings where a recognition and application of empathy can be established. This book, the contributions of the writers, and your leadership will make this possible. Have at it!

Thanks empathy!

– MIKEY KERIN

Contributors' Biographies

Shaykh Umar Al-Qadri: Chairperson of the Irish Muslim Peace & Integration Council and chief Imam at the Islamic Centre of Ireland.

Ella Anderson: BA in Law, Sociology and Political Science Graduate and a Youth Researcher with UNESCO.

Rachael Blackmore: Irish jockey, winner of Aintree Grand National 2021 and Cheltenham Gold Cup 2022.

Blindboyboatclub: Irish writer of fiction, podcasts and television.

Mark Brennan: Professor and UNESCO chair for Community, Leadership, and Youth Development at The Pennsylvania State University.

Bernadine Brady: Lecturer in the School of Political Science & Sociology and associate director of the UNESCO Child & Family Research Centre at the University of Galway.

Gillian Browne: Administrative assistant for UNESCO Child and Family Research Centre at the University of Galway.

Sarah-Anne Buckley: Head of the Department of History and senior research fellow at UNESCO Child and Family Research Centre at the University of Galway.

Seán Campbell: CEO of Foróige and a member of the National Children and Young People's Advisory Council which advises the Minister for Children, Equality, Disability, Integration and Youth.

Niamh Condon: Dysphagia chef, is the owner of Dining with Dignity Ltd, expert in dysphagia recipe practices, trainer, consultant, lecturer, guest speaker.

Mary Coughlan: Irish singer, songwriter and actress.

Michelle Darmody: Award-winning food writer, activist and researcher with extensive experience in food consultancy, which brings together food, creativity and sustainability.

Tara Dawson: Honours fourth year student studying a BA in Child, Youth and Family (Policy and Practice) at the University of Galway.

Catherine Denning: Theatre tutor, actor, voice over and community artist based in the west of Ireland. She currently works in Galway Community College of Further Education.

Louis de Paor: His most recent collections of poems are *Obair Bhaile* (2021) and *Grá Fiar/Crooked Love* (2022).

Emer Davitt: Lecturer with the School of Education at the University of Galway.

Brendan (Postdoctoral Researcher), **Eoin** (Youth Worker) and **Róisín** (Career Guidance Counseller) **Dolan** were born and raised in Galway City.

Pat Dolan: Professor and UNESCO Chair in Children Youth and Civic Engagement at the University of Galway.

Aisling Duffy: An eighteen-year-old student from Galway, who completed student work experience in the UNESCO Research Centre at the University of Galway.

Ashling Dunphy: Aged twenty-one, from Ballyneale, Carrick-on-Suir, County Tipperary. Currently studying applied social science community and youth work in Maynooth University.

Saoirse Egan: Proud Galway girl and sixth year student in Salerno, Galway.

Elaine Feeney: Writer and lecturer from the west of Ireland. Her latest novel is *As You Were* (2020)

Clodagh Finn: *Irish Examiner* columnist, journalist and author.

Eamonn Fitzgerald: Worked in construction, manufacturing and for the last twenty years in retail management.

Hugh Fitzmaurice is currently a Mind and Performance coach who runs his own coaching business, Claritycoach.ie. He has also worked with the University of Galway in piloting an Activating Social Empathy programme for secondary school students across the country.

Niamh Flynn is an educational psychologist and lecturer in the School of Education at the University of Galway.

Kiernan Forsyth is a retired postman and qualified volunteer football coach.

John Gaffey is a youth researcher and BA graduate in History, Celtic Studies and Creative Writing of University of Galway.

Ailbhe Greaney is currently an artist, lecturer and director of Photography with Video at the Belfast School of Art, Faculty of Arts, Humanities and Social Sciences, Ulster University. Born in Galway she has also lived in New York as a Fulbright and Aaron Siskind Memorial Scholar.

Marcus Hannick is a civil engineer MSc, BEng (Hons), business owner and executive director of Drex Corp in New York.

Róisín Hanley is a Royal Academy of Dance qualified ballet teacher and a graduate of BA Children's Studies at the University of Galway 2022.

Niamh Heery is a writer, director and community filmmaker from Dublin.

Tiernan Henry is an academic who lives and works in Galway.

President Michael D. Higgins is the ninth president of Ireland and was re-elected in 2018 to serve a second term. President Higgins has served at every level of public life, is a published poet and has published four books of essays and speeches.

Rita Ann Higgins was born and lives in Galway. She writes poems and plays. She has written two screenplays in Irish.

Kitty Holland is social affairs correspondent at *The Irish Times,* she has reported widely on social justice and human rights issues such as homelessness, drug addiction, poverty, women's rights, immigrants' rights, asylum seekers, domestic violence and LGBTQ rights.

Hozier is an Irish Grammy-nominated, award-winning multi-platinum singer and songwriter.

Ben Hughes is the head of Chaplaincy and Pastoral Care at the University of Galway, and the founder of the university's Seas Suas Bystander Intervention Programme.

Pat and John Hume worked as peace activists for many years in Northern Ireland. Committed to inclusion, non-violence and community building, they were central in the movement to peace and political agreement. John was awarded the Nobel peace prize. Written by Therese, Áine and Aidan Hume.

Kathy Hyland is the art therapist at the Galway and Mayo Hospice Foundation.

Pamela Joyce is a Galway native who presents the lunchtime show on Today FM from 12–2 p.m. Pamela has also written and starred in a number of RTÉ Player original series.

Nicola Joyce is a singer, musician and songwriter from Headford, Co. Galway. She is a member of folk group The Whileaways.

John Kelly has published two collections of poetry: *Notions* (2018) and *Space* (2022).

Mikey Kerin is a very social outgoing person, who is very patient. He likes to be kind, generous and helpful and is a team player.

Rabbi Zalman Lent is leader of the Dublin Hebrew Congregation and director of Chabad Ireland.

James Leonard is a team leader at Coolmine Drug and Alcohol Service, lecturer at University College Cork and host of *The Two Norries* podcast.

Marie Lohan is a staff nurse in the Emergency Department, Sligo University Hospital.

Timmy Long is co-host of *The Two Norries* podcast. He works in his own construction firm as a carpenter and co-manages a carwash and valeting business where the emphasis is to employ people in recovery and desistance from crime.

Neven Maguire is proprietor and head chef at MacNean House & Restaurant in Blacklion, Co Cavan. He is well known for his chart topping cookery books and is a regular radio and television broadcaster.

Tolu Makay an artist, singer and songwriter, actor, performer and mental health advocate.

Imelda May is a singer, songwriter, performer and poet who is one of Ireland's most celebrated female artists. Selling millions of records worldwide, Imelda is a Women's Rights Activist and released her first poetry book *A Lick & A Promise* (2022).

Martin McDonagh is a Foróige project worker with the Eastside Youth Service UBU in Ballybane, Galway.

Jack McDonough is a retired Chief United States Probation Officer and former deputy director of Youth Rehabilitative Services for the State of Delaware.

Kalyn McDonough is a post-doctoral fellow with the Partnership for Healthy Communities at the University of Delaware.

Mary McGill is a Media Studies lecturer, journalist and former Hardiman scholar at the University of Galway. Her first book, *The Visibility Trap: Sexism, Surveillance and Social Media* (2021).

Paul McGrath is a retired professional footballer.

Susan McKeown is a Grammy-winning singer-songwriter and producer, and the founder and director of Cuala Foundation.

Hugo MacNeill is a former Irish rugby international who went on to have a career in international business. He has worked with many not-for-profit organisations relating to North-South and British Irish relations and in recent years has worked with the Trinity Centre for People with Intellectual Disabilities.

Fr Peter McVerry, SJ, works with homeless people.

Cillian Murphy, actor and patron of the UNESCO Child and Family Research Centre, University of Galway.

Cathal Murray, Athlone native, is a radio presenter with RTÉ Radio 1, Ireland's public service broadcaster.

Ciara-Beth Ní Ghríofa is an autism advocate and UNESCO youth researcher, with an interest in how technology can be designed and used to improve the lives of people with disabilities. She's currently finishing her undergraduate degree in psychology and computing in UCC, and hopes to continue to work in a field.

Gary Nugent is a senior youth officer, Foróige, The National Youth Development Organisation.

Carl O'Brien is education editor of *The Irish Times.*

Brendan O'Connor is a journalist/broadcaster.

Uchechukwu Helen Ogbu is a doctoral researcher at the UNESCO Child and Family Research Centre, University of Galway and part-time development worker with Galway Volunteer Centre.

Rebecca O'Connor is a senior lecturer at the University of Limerick and is the Creative Arts Therapy Service lead, researcher and senior music therapist at the National Rehabilitation Hospital, Ireland.

Louise O'Neill is from Clonakilty, in West Cork. She is the award winning author of *Asking For It* (2015) and *Idol* (2022).

Rory O'Neill/Panti Bliss is a performer, writer, gender discombobulist and pub landlady. They live in Dublin with a dog, a cat, and a fella.

Joanne O'Riordan studied criminology in UCC and is only one of seven people in the world living with a rare physical disability known as total amelia.

Eamon O'Shea is an economist working at the University of Galway. His main research interests are ageing and dementia. He has played hurling for Tipperary at all levels and has coached and managed the Tipperary team in recent years.

Valerie Biden Owens is the first woman in US history to have run a presidential campaign – that of her brother, Joseph R.

Biden, Jr. Today, Valerie is chair of the Biden Institute at the University of Delaware and serves on the advisory board of the Beau Biden Foundation for the Protection of Children.

The Very Rev. Lynda Peilow is rector of St Nicholas' Collegiate church, Galway, Church of Ireland rector, ordained 1997. She is currently the Church of Ireland's Central Director of Ordinands, and has served in several hospital chaplaincy roles throughout her ministry.

Fiona Whelan Prine is president of Oh Boy Records, founded by her late husband, John Prine. Born and raised in Ireland, Fiona is the eldest of six daughters born to Donal and Mary Whelan. She also serves as founder and president of the newly established Hello in There Foundation.

Colin Regan is the community and health manager with the Gaelic Athletic Association. Previously a journalist/editor, he represented Leitrim and his club Melvin Gaels in Gaelic football.

Stephanie Roche, an Irish international footballer, played professionally in some of the top leagues in the world including WSL in England and NWSL in the US. Most recently has become a TV panellist for RTÉ Sports and Premier sports covering international, premier league and champions league football.

Matthew Shaw-Torkzadeh is a first year student at Newpark Comprehensive School in Dublin.

Charlotte Silke is a post-doctoral researcher with the UNESCO Child and Family Research Centre at the University of Galway.

Elaine and Alan Smith are both from Belfast. They met as students in 1974 and married in 1981, worked in Africa, then became involved in the establishment of integrated schools in Northern Ireland. Now retired. Elaine was a teacher of French and Spanish and Alan was UNESCO chair at Ulster University.

Mary Sugrue, a native of Cahersiveen, Co. Kerry, is chief executive of the Irish American Partnership, Boston, whose members honour and celebrate their Irish heritage by investing in Ireland's future.

The Edge is a musician, activist and founding member of U2.

Martina Venneman is a member of An Garda Síochána and is based in Co. Donegal, Ireland.

Dermot Whelan is a comedian, broadcaster, author, meditation teacher and public speaker.

Annie White is the senior research associate at the Fred Rogers Institute at Saint Vincent College, Latrobe, PA.

Dana Winters is executive director of the Fred Rogers Institute and a professor of Arts, Humanities, and Social Sciences at Saint Vincent College.